T0276870

Diagnosis and Treatment of Aneurysm

Diagnosis and Treatment of Aneurysm

Edited by **Lizzy Rattini**

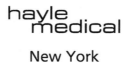

New York

Published by Hayle Medical,
30 West, 37th Street, Suite 612,
New York, NY 10018, USA
www.haylemedical.com

Diagnosis and Treatment of Aneurysm
Edited by Lizzy Rattini

Contents

Preface

This book aims to serve as an up-to-date resource guide for understanding aneurysm. As it discusses basic researches related to aneurysm. It focuses on the analysis and handling of abdominal and thoracic aortic aneurysms. It will be helpful for vascular and cardiothoracic experts, and also for readers involved in vascular medication. The book attempts to compile recent information and achievements in this field of science. The objective of this book is to help experts in carrying their researches forward and produce some fruitful outcomes. It thoroughly describes all the aspects of abdominal and splenial aneurysm.

Various studies have approached the subject by analyzing it with a single perspective, but the present book provides diverse methodologies and techniques to address this field. This book contains theories and applications needed for understanding the subject from different perspectives. The aim is to keep the readers informed about the progresses in the field; therefore, the contributions were carefully examined to compile novel researches by specialists from across the globe.

Indeed, the job of the editor is the most crucial and challenging in compiling all chapters into a single book. In the end, I would extend my sincere thanks to the chapter authors for their profound work. I am also thankful for the support provided by my family and colleagues during the compilation of this book.

Editor

Basic Research of Aneurysm

Biomechanics and FE Modelling of Aneurysm: Review and Advances in Computational Models

Simona Celi and Sergio Berti

Additional information is available at the end of the chapter

1. Introduction

Abdominal aortic aneurysm (AAA) disease is the 18th most common cause of death in all individuals and the 15th most common in individuals aged over 65 [48]. Clinical treatment for this disorder can consist of open surgical repair or, more recently, of minimally invasive endovascular repair procedures [71]. However, both clinical treatments present significant risks and, consequently, require specific patient selection. Given the risks of current repair techniques, during the course of an aneurysm it is important to determine when the risk of rupture justifies the risk of repair. In this scenario, how to determine the rupture risk of an aneurysm is still an open question. Currently, the trend in determining the severity of an AAA is to use the maximum diameter criterion. Unfortunately, this criterion is only a general rule and not a reliable indicator since small aneurysms can also rupture, as reported in autopsy studies, while many aneurysms can become very large without rupturing [16]. The maximum diameter criterion, in fact, is based on the law of Laplace that establish a linear relationship between diameter and wall stress. However, the law of Laplace is simply based on cylindrical geometries, where only one radius of curvature is involved, whereas aneurysms are complex structures, and therefore the law fails to predict realistic wall stresses. From a biomechanical point of view, rupture events occur when acting wall stresses exceed the tensile strength of the degenerated aortic abdominal (AA) wall. Biomechanics relates the function of a physiological system to its structure and its objective is to deduce the function of a system from its geometry, material properties and boundary conditions based on the balance laws of mechanics (e.g. conservation of mass, momentum and energy). Consequently, from a more general and extensive perspective, the stress state in a body is determined by several factors such as geometry, material properties, load and boundary conditions. In order to understand the capability to estimate the potential rupture risk, it is fundamental to capture the mechanical response of the aortic tissue and its changes during aneurysmal formation. In fact, while, to date, the precise pathogenesis of AAA is poorly understood, it is well known that this change significantly impact on the structure of the aortic wall and on its mechanical behavior.

This chapter will review the state of literature on the mechanical properties and modelling of AAA tissue and will present advanced computational models. The first part (Sec. 2) includes a description of the mechanical test currently used (2.1), the aortic mechanical properties (2.2) and a review of the literature on material constitutive equations (2.3) and geometrical models (2.4). To stress out the morphological complexity of the aortic segment, in Sec 3 the regional variations of material properties and wall thickness reported in literature form experimental investigations are reported. The second part (Sec. 4) describes our original contribution with a description of our Finite Element (FE) models and our probabilistic approach implemented into FE simulations to perform sensitivity analysis (Sec. 4.1). The main results are reported in Sec. 4.2 and discussed in detail in Sec. 5.

2. Review

In order to understand the biomechanical issues in the etiology and treatment of abdominal aortic aneurysms, it is important to understand the structures of the aortic wall and how they affect the mechanical response. Biological tissues are subject to the same balance laws of conservation of mass, momentum and energy of the classical engineering material. What distinguish biological tissues from materials of the field of classical engineering mechanics is their unique structure. Soft biological tissues, in fact, have a very complex structure that can be regarded as either *active* and *passive*. The active components arise from the activation of the smooth muscle cells while the passive response is governed primarily by the elastin and collagen fibres [15]. The distribution and the arrangement of the collagen fibres, in particular, have a significant influence on the mechanical properties due to they attribute anisotropic properties [49] to the tissue. Different studies have shown that this structural arrangement is very complex and varies according to the aortic segment (thoracic or abdominal) [20]. As well as being anisotropic, the material response of soft biological tissue is also highly non-linear.

2.1. Experimental test

To determine mechanical properties of AAA, studies have used both *in-vivo* "tests" and *ex-vivo/in-vitro* testing. As reported by Raghavan and da Silva [53], both of them offer advantages and disadvantages. In particular, in the first case the main difficult is to accurately determine the true force and the displacement distribution ascertaining stress-free configuration of the biological entity. On the other side, isolating samples may introduce as yet unknown changes to their behavior affecting the results of such tests. In vivo measurement are often performed by using imaging modality. By using ultrasound phase-locked echo-tracking, Lanne et al. [43] reported that the pressure-strain elastic modulus (E_p), Eq. 1, was higher on average and more widely dispersed in aneurysmal abdominal aorta compared to the non-aneurysmal aorta group. The E_p modulus was calculated based on the diameter (D_s, D_d) and pressure (P_s, P_d) at the systolic and diastolic values as follow:

$$E_p = D_p \frac{P_s - P_d}{D_s - D_d} \tag{1}$$

Using similar consideration, MacSweeney et al. [44] founded that E_p was higher in aneurysmal abdominal aorta compared to controls.

More recently, van't Veer et al. [75] estimated the compliance and distensibility of the AAA by means of simultaneous instantaneous pressure and volume measurements obtained with the magnetic resonance imaging (MRI). By using time resolved ECG-gated CT imaging data from 67 patients, Ganten et al. [27] found that the compliance of AAA did not differ between small and large lesions. In 2011 Molacek and co-authors [47] did not find any correlation between aneurysm diameter and distensibility of AAA wall and of normal aorta. However it is worth to notice that all these studies do not provide intrinsic mechanical properties of the tissue but more general extrinsic AAA behavior. As far as the *ex-vivo* testing, there are several types of mechanical tests that can be carried out on materials to obtain information on their mechanical behavior. Such tests include simple tension test, biaxial tension, conducted on thin samples of material, and extension/inflation test of thin-walled tubes.

Uniaxial test. Uniaxial extension testing is the simplest and most common of *ex-vivo* testing methods. Here, a rectangular planar sample is subjected to extension along its length at a constant displacement (or load) rate while the force (or the displacement) is recorded during extension. Under the assumption of incompressibility (zero changes of volume during the tensile test, Eq. 2) the recorded force-extension data are converted to stress/strain:

$$A_0 L_0 = AL \tag{2}$$

where A_0 and L_0 are the initial cross sectional area and the initial length while A and L are the values in the current configuration. Interested reader can refer to Di Puccio et al. [19] for a recent review on the incompressibility assumption on soft biological tissue.

Biaxial test. Due to the presence of the collagen fibers, the uniaxial testing is not sufficient for highlighting the aorta tissue and the stress distribution does not fully conform to physiological conditions. Therefore, biaxial tension tests should be performed. During biaxial test, an initial square thin sheet of material is stress normally to both edges. Even if, theoretically, the biaxial test are not sufficient to fully characterized anisotropic materials, [40, 50] they are able to capture additional information regarding the mechanical behavior of the specimens with respect to uniaxial one. By contrast, biaxial tests provides a complete characterization of the material properties for isotropic material. To some extent soft biological tissues can be considered as isotropic within certain limitation, however, in their general formulation, they respond anisotropically under loads. Figure 1 depicts as example the mechanical test and response of a soft tissue under uniaxial (a) and biaxial (b) test.

As we can observe, a distinctive mechanical characteristic of soft tissue in tension tests is its initial flat response and relatively large extensions followed by an increased stiffening at higher extension. As it is well known, this behavior is the result of collagen fibres recruitment as proposed by Roach and Burton [61]. The non-linear stress strain curve arises from the phenomenon of the fibres recruitment. As the material is stretched, the fibres gradually become uncrimped and become more aligned with the direction of applied load.

The results of uniaxial and biaxial tests are used to characterize the mechanical behavior of soft tissue under investigation. Due to the large deformation that characterizes this type of tissue, from a mathematical point of view, a Strain Energy Function (SEF) denoted by W is introduced. The Cauchy stress tensor (σ) is calculated as:

$$\sigma = J^{-1} \mathbf{F} \frac{\partial W}{\partial \mathbf{F}} \tag{3}$$

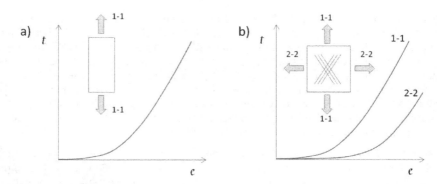

Figure 1. Schematic of uniaxial (a) and biaxial (b) test and curves. The t value is a rappresentative tension value and e a typical extension dimension.

where $\mathbf{F}$ is the deformation gradient tensor, defined as $\mathbf{F} = \partial \mathbf{x}/\partial \mathbf{X}$, i.e. the derivative of the current position $\mathbf{x}$ as regards to the initial position $\mathbf{X}$ during a deformation process and J is the determinant of $\mathbf{F}$. Under the assumption of incompressibility ($J=1$), the SEF is split in a volumetric (W_{vol}) and isochoric (W_{isoch}) component. In case of uniaxial test we have:

$$\sigma_{11} = \lambda_{11} \frac{\partial W_{isoch}}{\partial \lambda_{11}} \tag{4}$$

where λ_{11} is the stretch in the 1-1 direction (see Fig. 1 (a)). For biaxial test both components can be calculated:

$$\sigma_{\theta\theta} = \lambda_{\theta\theta} \frac{\partial W_{isoch}}{\partial \lambda_{\theta\theta}} \tag{5}$$

$$\sigma_{zz} = \lambda_{zz} \frac{\partial W_{isoch}}{\partial \lambda_{zz}} \tag{6}$$

Equations 5-6 represent the stress components used in the follow sections. With respect to Fig. 1 direction 1-1 and 2-2 are now defined as the circumferential $\sigma_{\theta\theta}$ and the axial σ_{zz} ones, respectively.

2.2. Mechanical properties of healthy and pathological aortic tissue

AAA development is multifactorial phenomenon. A mechanism postulated for AAA formation focuses on inflammatory processes where macrophages recruitment leads to MMP production and elastase release. The biomechanical change associated with enzymatic degradation of structural proteins suggests that AAA expansion is primarily related to elastolysis [21]: a decreasing quadratic relationship was found between elastin concentration and diameter for normal aortas and for pathological increasing diameter [65]. Despite universal recognition of the importance of wall mechanics in the natural history of AAAs [2, 38, 81], there are few detailed studies of the mechanical properties.

Early studies focused on simple uniaxial tests. He and Roach [32] obtained rectangular specimen strips during surgical resection of eight AAA patients and subjected them to uniaxial extension tests up to a pre-defined maximum load rather than until failure. They showed that the stress-strain behavior of AAA tissue was non-linear. Later, in two reports,

Vorp et al. [82] and Raghavan et al. [57] reported on uniaxial extension testing of strips harvested from the anterior midsection of 69 AAA. The specimens were extended until failure. In most cases, the rectangular specimens' length was in the axial orientation, but in a small population, they were oriented circumferentially. Results have found that aneurysmal tissue is substantially weaker and stiffer than normal aorta [18, 57, 70].

To date, the most complete data on both the biaxial mechanical behavior of aorta and AAAs comes from Vande Geest et al. [76, 77]. The source of these specimens becomes from AAA ventral tissue available during the open surgical repair of unruptured lesions. They reported biaxial mechanical data for AAA (26 samples) and normal human AA as a function of age: less than 30, between 30 and 60 and over 60 years of age. In particular Vande Geest and co-workers confirmed that the aortic tissue becomes less compliant with age and that AAA tissue is significantly stiffer than normal abdominal aortic tissue, Figure 2.

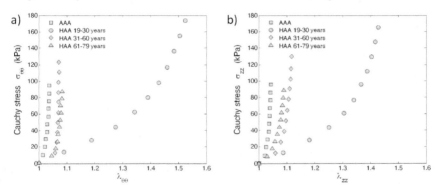

Figure 2. Stress-stretch plot comparing the equibiaxial response for AAA and HAA for four patient groups, for circumferential direction (a) and axial direction (b). Modified from [22].

The specimen was subjected to force-controlled testing with varying prescribed forces between the two orthogonal directions. A CCD camera was used to track the displacement of markers forming a 5x5 mm square placed on the specimen. It is worth to stress out that the use of optical extensometer (markers tracking with CCD camera) is fundamental to measure the deformation during test avoiding the potential tissue slippage from the clamps. Figure 3 depicts a representative biaxial stress-stretch data for healthy (a-b) and pathological (c-d) samples considering three different tension ratios ($T_\theta : T_z$) equal to 1:1 , 0.75:1 and 1:0.75.

2.3. Material models

Equations that characterize a material and its response to applied loads are called constitutive relations since they describe the gross behavior resulting from the internal constitution of a material. Constitutive modelling of vascular tissue is an active field of research and numerous descriptions have been reported. Constitutive models for biological tissues can be established following a so-called phenomenological or structural approach. The first type of formulation [14, 26, 36, 73] does not take into account any histological constituents and attempt to describe the global mechanical behavior of the tissue without referring to its underlying microstructure. The phenomenological approach is commonly used but has led to a number of difficulties in describing the mechanical behavior of tissues. Among phenomenological

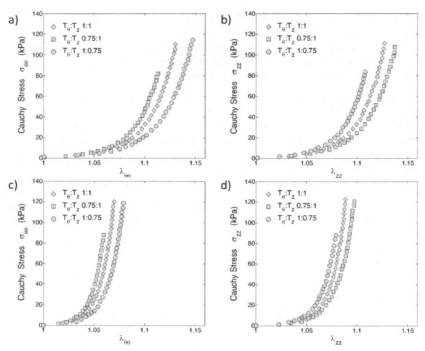

Figure 3. Experimental biaxial data for both healthy (a-b) and pathological (c-d) samples with different tension ratio. Open diamonds, 1 : 1; open squares, 0.75 : 1 and open circles, 1 : 0.75. Modified from [9].

SEFs, Vande Geest and co-authors [77] found that a constitutive functional form used earlier by Choi and Vito [12], Equation 7, would best suit their experimental data:

$$W_{isoch} = b_0 \left(e^{\frac{1}{2} b_1 E_{\theta\theta}^2} + e^{\frac{1}{2} b_2 E_{zz}^2} + e^{\frac{1}{2} b_3 E_{\theta\theta} E_{zz}} - 3 \right) \tag{7}$$

where b_0, b_1, b_2 and b_3 are the material parameters and $E_{\theta\theta}$ and E_{zz} are the components of the Green-strain tensor (Eq. 8) defined as follows:

$$\mathbf{E} = \frac{1}{2} \left(\mathbf{C} - \mathbf{I} \right) = \frac{1}{2} \left(\mathbf{FF}^T - \mathbf{I} \right) \tag{8}$$

where $\mathbf{I}$ is the identity matrix and $\mathbf{C}$ is the right Cauchy-Green strain tensor.

Alternatively, structural constitutive descriptions [5, 28, 34, 35] overcome this limitation and integrate histological and mechanical information of the arterial wall. In particular, the contributions of constitutive cells, fibers and networks of elements are added together to depict the whole tissue behavior. The structural-based approach has become common with the advent of microstructural imaging methods [64, 80]. In fact, soft biological tissues have a very complex microstructure, consisting of many different components and including elastin fibres, collagen fibres, smooth muscle cells and extracellular matrix.

The same experimental data obtained by vande Geest et al. [77] were then fitted by using an invariant based constitutive equation with two fibre families (2FF) by Basciano et al. [5], Eq.

9, and Rodriguez et al. [62, 63], Eq. 10.

$$W_{isoch} = \alpha \left(\bar{I}_1 - 3\right)^2 + \beta \left(\bar{I}_4 - 1\right)^6 + \gamma \left(\bar{I}_6 - 1\right)^6 \tag{9}$$

$$W_{isoch} = C_1 \left(\bar{I}_1 - 3\right) + \sum_{i=3}^{4} \frac{k_1^i}{2k_2^i} \left(e^{k_2^i \left((1-\rho)(\bar{I}_1 - 3)^2 + \rho(\bar{I}_4 - I_0)^2\right)} - 1\right) \tag{10}$$

where $\bar{I}_1$ is the first invariant of the isochoric portion of the right Cauchy-Green stretch tensor (Eq. 11) and $\bar{I}_4$ and $\bar{I}_6$ are mixed invariants of the isochoric portion of the right Cauchy-Green deformation tensor (Eq. 12-13), introduced from embedded fibers [6, 33, 69].

$$\bar{I}_1 = tr\bar{C} \tag{11}$$

$$\bar{I}_4 = \mathbf{a}_0 \cdot \bar{C} \, \mathbf{a}_0 \tag{12}$$
$$\bar{I}_6 = \mathbf{b}_0 \cdot \bar{C} \, \mathbf{b}_0 \tag{13}$$

where $\mathbf{a}_0$, $\mathbf{b}_0$ are the direction of the fibers as reported in Figure 4(a-b). In Eq. 9, α is the coefficients for the isotropic part while β and γ for the anisotropic component. In the same manner, in Eq. 10, C_1 is a stress-like material parameter for the purely elastin contribute, and k_j^i are material parameters corresponding to the fibers ($k_1^3 = k_1^4$ and $k_2^3 = k_2^4$). The parameter $\rho \in [0;1]$ is a (dimensionless) measure of anisotropy, $I_0 > 1$ is dimensionless parameters regarded as the initial crimping of the fibers (Fig. 4(b)).

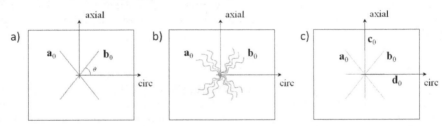

Figure 4. Collagen fiber orientation ($\mathbf{a}_0$, $\mathbf{b}_0$) in a square specimen of tissue for the 2FF model (a), the 2FF model with dispersion (b) and for the 4FF model (c). Note the crimp and fibres dispersion in case (b) and the two additional fibre family ($\mathbf{c}_0$, $\mathbf{d}_0$) in (c).

A constitutive relation based on four fibres family (4FF) (Fig. 4(c)) was proposed by Baek et al. [4], including two additionally fibres family (in longitudinal and circumferential direction, [86]), Equation 14:

$$W_{isoch} = \frac{c}{2} \left(\bar{I}_1 - 3\right) + \sum_{i=1}^{4} \frac{c_1^i}{4c_2^i} \left(e^{c_2^i \left(\bar{I}_4^i - 1\right)^2} - 1\right) \tag{14}$$

where c, c_1^i and c_2^i are material parameters for this specific SEF. Ferruzzi et al. [22] assumed that diagonal families of collagen were regarded as mechanically equivalent, hence $c_1^3 = c_1^4$, $c_2^3 = c_2^4$. By fitting the biaxial data, the model parameter associated with the isotropic term decreased with increasing age for AA specimens and decreased markedly for AAA specimens [22, 31]. These finding are in good agreement with histopathological results of reduced elastin in ageing [30, 51] and AAAs, e.g. [32, 60].

For all models, the diagonal fibres are accounted for by $\mathbf{a}_0 = -\mathbf{b}_0$; in the 4FF model, axial ($\mathbf{c}_0$) and circumferential ($\mathbf{d}_0$) fibres are fixed at 90° and 0°, respectively.

Among the variety of constitutive equations reported in literature, the most significant difference in structural formulation were included by Holzapfel group [62] and by Baek and co-authors [4]. For a more detailed analysis on the effect of this assumption and a comparison between the two constitutive model, interested reader can refer to [17]. It is worth to stress out that, as observed by Zeinali-Davarani and co-authors [87], in parameter estimation, the larger number of parameters for a model provides more flexibility and generally gives better fitting, i.e., decreases the residual error. A common assumption in all previous models is to assume the same fibers distribution and mechanical response throughout the thickness. More recently Schriefl et al. [66] has observed that in the case of the intima layer, due to the higher fibers dispersion, the number of fiber families varying from two to four. However, not all intimas investigated had more than two fiber families while two prominent fibers families were always visible. The number of fiber families equal to two was previously reported by Haskett et al. [31] by analyzing 207 aortic samples.

Finally, it is worth to notice that it is fundamental to define a constitutive model and its material constants over some specific range, from experiments that replicate conditions (physiological or pathological), [17], in order to provide more accurate response. In fact all constitutive formulation are based on specific assumptions and hypotheses. The complexities of the artery wall poses several new conceptual and methodological challenges in the cardiovascular biomechanics. There exist several recent frameworks, in fact, to develop theories of arterial growth and remodeling (G&R) of soft tissues. Interested reader can refer to a more complete and detailed review by Humphrey and Rajagopal [38, 39] and in [41]. However, in this study, we restrict our attention to structural based formulations to emphasize their particular effects.

2.4. Geometrical model

By using Finite Element analyses, Fillinger et al. [23] showed that peak wall stress is a more reliable parameter than maximum transverse diameter in predicting potential rupture event. These findings appear to be supported by the results obtained by Venkatasubramaniam et al. [79], who indicated that the location of the maximum wall stress correlates well with the site of rupture and, additionally, by the observation that AAA formation is accompanied by an increase in wall stress [55, 83], and a decrease in wall strength [84]. Simulation on 3D patient-specific models are aimed to analyze the distribution of the wall stress to estimate the rupture risk during the evolution of the pathology [23], the effect of the thrombus [29, 85] or calcification [42, 45, 68] on the peak stress. Integration of geometry data with solid modelling is used for estimation of vessel wall distension, strain and stress patterns. Studies, to date, have typically used 3D geometries usually obtained from computer tomography (CT) [52] or MRI [7] scans or have used simplified morphologies [17, 62]. Figure 5 reports as example the phases from a CT reconstruction. However, both approaches present some limitations. In particular, it is worth pointing out that 3D simulations are not fully patient-specific models but only based on 3D patient-specific geometries while the material properties are assumed as mean population values due to the difficulty of assessing *in-vivo* material properties. Consequently, to date, no fully patient-specific model has been performed. Additionally, due to the complexity of the structure and the high computational cost required by patient-specific models, sensitivity analyses have not been performed on 3D real geometries, and only univariate investigations have been performed on idealized shapes, to estimate the influence of a single parameter on the whole stress map [63].

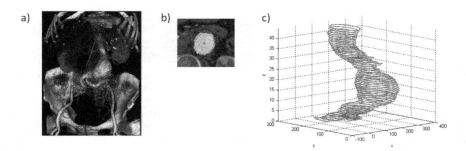

Figure 5. Example of AAA (a), segmentation of a CT cross section (b) and 3D reconstruction of a AAA (c), from [10].

3. Regional variations in wall thickness and material properties

As reported in previous section, starting from the observation that most AAAs are characterized by a complex not axisymmetric geometries a growing amount of literature has been published on the influence of the geometrical features. However one limitation in all the studies published so far is a constant wall thickness and homogeneous material assumed in the FE models.

Wall thickness. While the segmentation of the arterial lumen is a well established technique and has been performed with different modalities in living subjects, the segmentation of the wall and its connective components is not a feasible process due to the low contrast between the wall and the surrounding tissues. The conventional imaging techniques, in fact, do not provide sufficient spatial resolution to assess the wall thickness measurement and variant *in-vivo.*

During the AAA formation the artery wall is subjected to the remodelling process [77] and, as a consequence, the ratio between AA and AAA wall thickness changes. Di Martino et al. [18] noted a significant difference in wall thickness between ruptured and elective AAAs (3.6±0.3 mm vs 2.5±0.1 mm, respectively). By comparing the wall thickness between healthy and pathological samples, Vande Geest et al. [77] reported that the mean measured thickness values were 1.49±0.11 and 1.32±0.08 mm for the AA and AAA specimens, respectively. In all these studies, samples were measured only in the anterior area and consequently no information regarding regional variation between ventral and dorsal was reported. Thubrikar et al. [70] obtained five whole unruptured AAA specimens during surgical resection. Raghavan et al. [54] performed similar measures on three unruptured and one ruptured AAA, harvested as a whole during necropsy. More recently Celi et al. [10] performed measurements on 12 harvested unrupture ascending segments. In Table 1, the main results of these experimental measures are reported for both anterior and posterior region (mean±sd).

It is worth to notice that the thickness distribution seems to be opposite of that in the normal abdominal aorta where the wall is thicker than the posterior wall in 64% of cases [74].

From the computational point of view, in literature only few authors have investigated the effect on wall thickness reduction. Scotti et al. [67] used a non uniform wall thickness in an

N. of samples	District	$Thk_{anterior}$ (mm)	$Thk_{posterior}$ (mm)	Ref
5	AAA	2.09±0.51	2.73±0.46	[70]
4	AAA	2.25±0.37	2.34±0.48	[54]
12	aTAA	1.63±0.48	2.18±0.35	[10]

Table 1. Wall thickness measurements, reported in literature, categorized by circumferential location as anterior and posterior

idealized isotropic model to performed FSI simulations. Their results show that the models with a non uniform wall thickness have a maximum wall stress nearly four times that of a uniform one. Starting from experimental measurement on 12 human harvested ascending aortic samples, Celi et al. [10] developed structural 3D models of ascending AAA by including wall thickness regional variation between dorsal and ventral areas.

Material properties. As far as the material properties, to date, different behavior has funded between healthy (HAA) and pathological samples. However, due to the lack of sufficient biaxial data, a full characterization in regional variations are not provided (in circumferential direction in particular), and mechanical tests have been performed mainly in the ventral area where the bulge was formed. As well as the material properties change during the AAA progression, also the wall strength value changes. This aspect plays a fundamental role in the rupture phenomenon. In fact, the concept is that AAA rupture follows the basic principles of material failure; i.e., an aneurysm ruptures when the mural stresses or deformation meets an appropriate failure criterion. In the filed of the classical mechanics, this concept is defined by means of the potential rupture risk (RPI) parameter and quantify as the ratio of local wall stress to local wall strength:

$$RPI = \frac{local\ stress}{local\ strength} \tag{15}$$

In the same manner the safety factor (SF) can be used as the inverse of the RPI.

Thubrikar et al. [70] performed uniaxial tensile tests in both longitudinal and circumferential direction, on samples from five aneurysms. To study the regional variation they obtained samples from anterior, lateral (without distinction between left and right side) and posterior regions. In this study, however, authors did not perform tests until failure and they recorded the yield stress to define the initial point of a permanent damage. Thubrikar et al. observed that in both directions, the yield stress was greater in the lateral region with respect to the anterior and the posterior region, Figure 6(a). Experimental values regarding ultimate stress were reported by Raghavan et al. [54], Figure 6(b). They cut multiple longitudinally oriented rectangular specimen strips at various locations from three unruptured AAA and one ruptured AAA for a total of 48 strips. Samples were tested uniaxially until failure. They observed that the failure tension (ultimate) of specimen strips varied regionally from 55 kPa (near the rupture site) to 423 kPa at the undilated neck. However they report that there was no perceptible pattern in failure properties along the circumference.

Using multiple linear regression, Vande Geest et al. [78] proposed a mathematical model to estimate the wall strength by including several mixed parameters such as the gender, the presence of the intraluminal thrombus (ILT) and the family history. The final statistical model for local Cauchy wall strength (Eq. 16, dimension in kPa) was given by:

$$\sigma_u = 719 - 379\left(ILT^{\frac{1}{2}} - 0.81\right) - 156\left(D_{NORM} - 2.46\right) - 213\,HIST + 193\,SEX \tag{16}$$

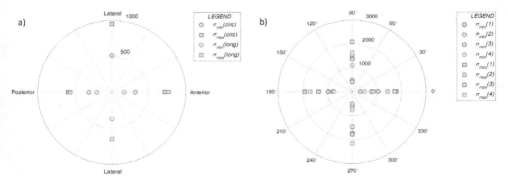

Figure 6. Yield stress in circumferential (upper side) and longitudinal (lower side) direction from [70] (a). Failure stress by circumferential location as anterior (0°), left (90°), posterior (180°) and right (270°) regions from [54] (b).

where $ILT^{\frac{1}{2}}$ is the square root of the ILT thickness whose units, D_{NORM} is a dimensionless parameter for local normalized diameter, HIST is a dimensionless binary variable (1/2 for positive family history, -1/2 for no family history), and SEX is a dimensionless binary variable for gender (1/2 for males, -1/2 for females). Table 2 depicts some examples of the effect of the coefficients of Eq. 16 by varing the gender and the ILT thickness.

Case	ILT (cm)	D_{NORM}	HIST	SEX	σ_u (kPa)
1	0	3.9	0.5	0.5	917.71
2	0	3.9	0.5	-0.5	598.35
3	1	3.9	0.5	-0.5	219.35

Table 2. Effect of the gender (case 1 vs. case 2) and of ILT thickness (case 2 vs. case 3) on the wall strength by using Eq. 16.

As we can notice the presence of the ILT decreases significantly the σ_u of about 63%. However, it is worth to notice that Eq. 16 describes local variation of the wall strength only in terms of normalized diameter and ILT thickness. Indeed Fillinger et al. [24] report that aneurysms likely rupture at stresses of 450 kPa or lower.

4. Finite element analyses

In order to get some indications on how regional variation of wall thickness and material properties affect the wall stress, two different FE models were developed. The first case describes a simplified model where an isotropic SEF has been adopted [56]. The tissue was described as homogeneous and consequently no distinction between healthy and pathological tissues was modeled. The second model introduces anisotropy and material regional variation to obtain more realistic simulations. For this last model, three different regions were considered and characterized with specific anisotropic SEFs: healthy material for the necks (HAA), pathological for the anterior bulge (AAA) and pathological for the posterior (AHA). Due to no data were available for the posterior region, a simple data manipulation was applied to define the new AHA pathological dataset starting from AAA experimental data as previously described in [9]. Figure 7 depicts the anisotropic dataset for the three rappresentative materials. As we can observe, the AHA dataset is able to reproduce an intermediate mechanical behavior between full healthy and pathological material.

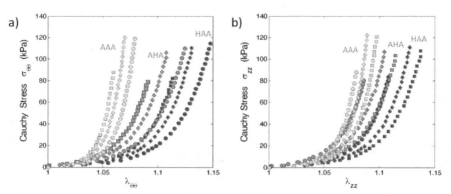

Figure 7. Example of HAA and AAA material models and virtual dataset (AHA) adopted for the transition region.

Both FE models are characterized by a wall thickness reduction in longitudinal and circumferential direction. For the necks, a wall thickness value equal to 1.8 mm was used while reduction of 30% and 50% was applied for the ventral area and of 20% for the dorsal one. Aneurysm shapes were defined as idealized 3D geometries with circular cross sections. Meridian lines describing the interior surface were based on a SZ-shaped function reported in Equation 17:

$$z(r) = \begin{cases} R_0 & 0 \leq z \leq a \\ 2(R_{AAA} - R_0)\left(\frac{z-a}{b-a}\right)^2 + R_0 & a < z \leq \frac{a+b}{2} \\ (R_{AAA} - R_0) - 2\left(\frac{z-b}{b-a}\right)^2 + R_0 & \frac{a+b}{2} < z \leq b \\ R_{AAA} & b < z \leq \frac{L}{2} \end{cases} \tag{17}$$

where the parameter a and b locate the extremes of the slope portion of the curve. Due to symmetry only one-half of the profile is reported. Geometrical profiles are reported in Fig. 8.

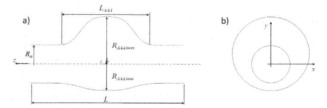

Figure 8. Lateral (a) and frontal (b) view of an asymmetrical aneurysmatic shape.

where where R_a is the radius of the healthy artery, $R_{AAA|max}$ is the maximum radius of the aneurysm in the ventral region, $R_{AAA|min}$ is the maximum radius of the aneurysm in the dorsal site. L (equal to 80 mm) defines the length of the abdominal vessel and L_{AAA} is the length of the aneurysmatic area. Figure 9(a) depicts an example of meshed asymmetric aneurysm with indication of the three anisotropic materials (in accordance with Fig. 7, while in Figure 9(b)) transversal cross section at the maximum diameter is reported with indication of circumferential wall thickness reduction.

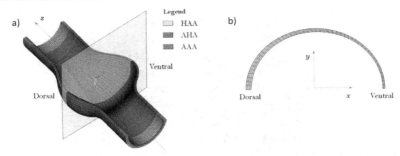

Figure 9. Example of asymmetric aneurysm and assignment of local material properties (a) and transversal cross section (b) with a wall thickness reduction of 50% and 20% in the ventral and dorsal region respectively.

For the constitutive equations for both healthy and pathological tissue, an invariant-based anisotropic polynomial SEF was chosen, as reported in Eq. 18. The material coefficients were calculated by using a specific weighted non-linear regression procedure implemented in Matlab and based on the Levenberg-Marquardt algorithm.

$$W_{isoch} = \sum_{i=1}^{3} a_i \left(\bar{I}_1 - 3\right)^i + 2 \sum_{j=2}^{6} b_j \left(\bar{I}_4 - 1\right)^j \tag{18}$$

Aneurysms were inflated applying a uniform inner pressure of 16 kPa, corresponding to the nominal value of peak systolic pressure. The ends of the vessels were left free to move in the radial direction.

4.1. Sensitivity analysis

To evaluate the sensitivity of the maximum stress state with respect to geometrical features, sensitivity and multivariate analyzes were also carried out by means of ANSYS Probabilistic Design Toolbox. This type of investigation presents two main advantages: the spread of the response of the output variables can be found, and it is possible to define the parameters that mainly influence the response of the system, for further details see [3, 46, 58]. Correlation coefficients are used as a measure of the strength of the relationship between input parameter and output measure.

In this study, analyzes were performed using the Monte Carlo method, in which the correlations between input and output variables are defined in a completely statistical way. In order to reduce the number of samples, the Latin Hypercube technique, instead of a direct sampling, was adopted. The effectiveness of these procedures was previously tested by Celi [8] and Celi et al. [11]. In order to study the effect of the AAA geometry on the distribution of the wall stresses, we introduced three dimensionless geometrical parameters:

$$F_R = \frac{R_{AAA}}{R_a}; \quad F_L = \frac{L_{AAA}}{R_{AAA}}; \quad F_{sym} = \frac{R_{AAA|min} - R_a}{R_{AAA|max} - R_a}; \quad F_{thk} = \frac{thk_0 - thk_{min}}{thk_0} 100 \tag{19}$$

The parameter F_R defines the ratio between the maximum AAA radius and the healthy arterial radius, F_L defines the ratio between the length of the aneurysm and the maximum AAA radius, while $F_{sym} \in [0,1]$ is a measure of the aneurysmal eccentricity. The extreme cases $F_{sym}=1$ and $F_{sym}=0$ define the symmetrical situation and the most asymmetric geometry, respectively. Table 3 summarizes the FE analyses performed in this study.

Parameter	Definition	Distribution	Range
F_R	Dilatation ratio	uniform	1.5-3
F_L	Shape factor	uniform	1.5-4
F_{sym}	Symmetry factor	uniform	0-1
F_{thk}	Thickness ratio	uniform	0-50

Table 3. Range of the geometric parameters defining the aneurysmal shape.

Model	Thk	N. of materials	Type of Material	Type of Analysis
Iso_1	variable	1 (AAA)	Iso	Det./Prob.
$Aniso_1$	variable	1 (AAA)	Aniso	Det.
$Aniso_3$	variable	3 (AAA, AHA, HAA)	Aniso	Det.

Table 4. Scheme of the simulations performed in this study.

4.2. Results

Fitting procedure. The results of the best fit procedures for the anisotropic SEFs are reported in Figure 10. For all models very good results were obtained and, as a metric of the goodness of fit, the root mean square of the fitting error were computed: $R^2=0.992$, $R^2=0.992$ and $R^2=0.983$ from healthy to pathological tissue, respectively.

Table 5 lists the parameters values for the HAA, AHA and AAA models. The angle θ represents the embedded fiber orientations, as illustrated in Fig. 4(a).

Model	a_1	a_3	a_3	b_4	b_5	b_6	θ	R^2
HAA	2.503	1.641	896.714	3.467	1.564	102.677	45.510	0.992
AHA	12.194	40.869	2166.994	2.483	41.883	64.650	52.199	0.992
AAA	1.5	0.1	4966.781	54.381	3856.291	4997.367	45.989	0.983

Table 5. Coefficients for the models for the three SEFs. Vales in kPa

Thus, the new models adequately reproduce the experimental data sets for HAA, AHA and AAA tissues using only one SEF with six parameters per model. Figure 10(c-f-i) points out the changes in the anisotropic effect by increasing the pathological response of a tissue from healthy to aneurysmatic state.

FE simulations. Distributions of the circumferential stresses for the isotropic and anisotropic models for three different values of F_{thk} are shown in Fig. 11. It can be observed that for all models and geometries, the maximum stress is localized in the interior wall surface and in the proximity of the minor radius of curvature, due to the geometrical effect of the curvature itself, and that there exists a stress gradient through the aneurysm wall thickness. As expected, the isotropic model underestimates the peak stress value of about 40%, 38%, 42% with respect to the 2FF homogeneous anisotropic model, Fig. 11(d-e-f), of about 44%, 40%, 43% with respect to the 2FF heterogeneous model, Fig. 11(g-h-i). By focusing our attention on the anisotropic

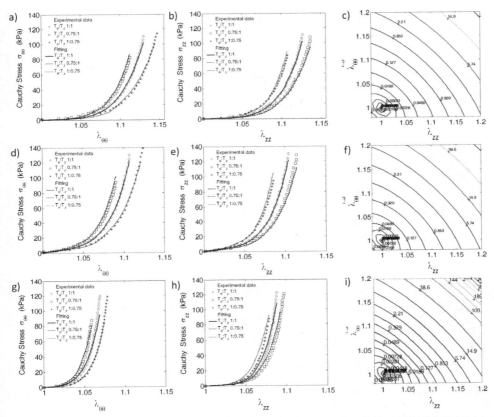

Figure 10. Representative stress-stretch data and fitting results for an HAA (a-b), AHA (d-e) and AAA (g-h) in circumferential and axial direction, see Fig. 7. The isolines of the SEFs for all models are reported in (c), (f) and (i).

models, as we can observe, the 2FF heterogeneous models present the highest maximum stress values due to the presence of the additional two material (HAA and AHA). The effect of these materials is to increase deformation in both radial and axial directions of the ventral and dorsal regions by changing, as a consequence, the local curvature.

As far as the stress gradient, Figure 12 depicts the transmural circumferential stress for model $Aniso_1$ and $Aniso_3$ for the two extreme cases of constant wall thickness and of maximum reduction. In the bulge area, Fig. 12(a), models $Aniso_1$ and $Aniso_3$ present the same stress gradient behavior due to the use of the same material (AAA). The effect of the wall thickness reduction is an increase of about 30% in the bulge region where the maximum diameter is reached. In the dorsal region, Fig. 12(b) the wall thickness reduction increases the maximum stress of about 8% for both models, while, the combined effect of the wall thickness reduction and different material produces an increase of about 21%. As far as the multivariate analysis, under the assumption of a constant wall thickness, the peak stress, is primarily affected by F_R, while if the wall thickness reduction in the bulge (F_{thk}) is considered, F_{thk} plays the main role.

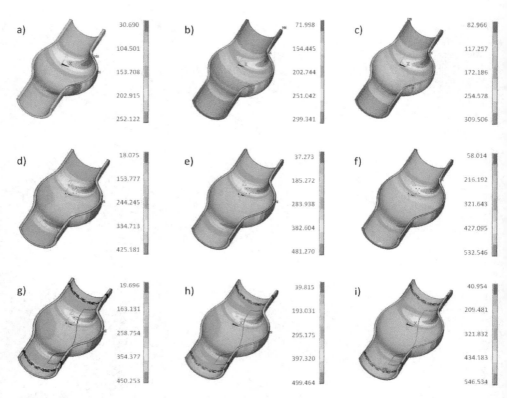

Figure 11. Contour plots of the circumferential stress for model Iso_1 (a-c), $Aniso_1$ (d-f) and $Aniso_3$ (g-i) with progressive wall thickness reduction. Constant wall *thk* (a,d,g), reduction of 30% and 20% (b,e,h) and reduction of 50% and 20% (c,f,i) in ventral and dorsal area. Stress in kPa.

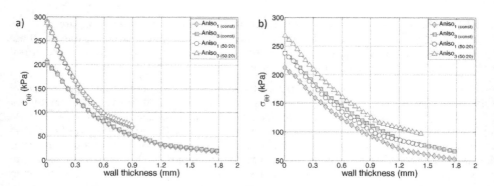

Figure 12. Stress gradient (kPa) in the ventral (a) and dorsal (b) area for the anisotropic models by considering constant wall thickness and the reduction of 50% and 20% in ventral and dorsal area.

Moreover, the same stress value is obtained both in fusiform aneurysm with critical dimension ($F_{thk} \simeq 2.5$) and in saccular with $F_{thk} \simeq 2$, see Figure 13(a). Including the wall thickness variation in the multivariate analyses points out the importance of these parameters. Figure 13(b) depicts the correlation coefficients (C.C.) for each input variable: the stresses increase as the diameter increases, but decrease as the thickness increases. Additionally, shorter models had higher wall stress.

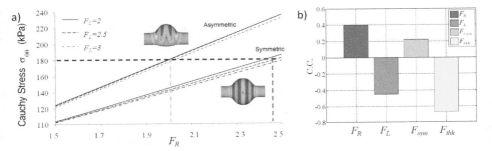

Figure 13. Maximum circumferential stresses as a function of F_R and F_L parameters (a) and correlation coefficients (C.C.) for each geometrical parameters (b).

5. Discussion and conclusion

In the first part of this work a literature survey on AAA biomechanics is reported by including several aspects from experimental test to constitutive model formulations. In the second part our FE models are presented, aimed at simulating and enhancing the computational study of the aneurismatic pathology. With respect to previous works, a more realistic type of AAA, even if idealized, was considered defined by means of regional variation of wall thickness and material properties. Notwithstanding many important findings from prior finite element stress analyses, all models are limited by the assumption of material homogeneity and constant wall thickness, e.g. [17, 55, 59, 62, 63]. Starting from the principle that intramural cells seek to remodel the arterial wall in order to maintain and to restore stresses towards homeostatic values, the material and geometrical properties must vary from region to region. This concept is the base of the remodeling phenomena as suggest by Humphrey [37]. In order to include material regional variation, in this work, we have introduced a simplified form of the stored energy function (Equation 18), motivated directly by microstructural information on two collagen fiber families [66]. This constitutive form fits well (e.g. mean R^2 of about 0.9) healthy and pathological available human biaxial data without complexity. Our SEF, in fact, is able to cope the progressive decrease in the elastin contribute (associated with the isotropic contribution attributed to an elastin-dominated amorphous matrix [34]) and increase in the anisotropic effects (associated with the predominant families of collagen fibers). The decrease of the elastin from heathy to pathological state as well as the increase of anisotropy are reported in Figure 14 where the isotropic (W_{iso}) and anisotropic (W_{aniso}) components of the SEF for HAA and AAA models are reported.

The present nonlinear regression focused not only on the estimating global best-fit values of model parameters suitable for performing stress analyses, but also on their effect in terms of energy behavior and changes from heathy to pathological tissue (Figure 10(c-i)). In

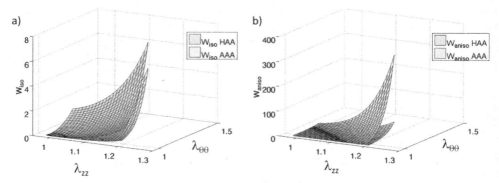

Figure 14. Isotopic (a) and anisotropic (b) component of the SEF reported in Eq. 18 for healthy (HAA) and pathological (AAA) tissue.

parallel to the marked decrease in the isotropic stored energy for AAA tissues (as describe above), we can observed an increase of stiffness capturing the observed biaxial reduction in extensibility/distensibility in particular in the circumferential direction (see Fig. 10(g)). As mention in Sec. 1, in current clinical practise, the aortic diameter is the main feature that is used to predict the risk of rupture. The more reliable quantification of the rupture risk is provided by the RPI parameter of Eq. 15 (and similar), however, which stress (principal stress, circumferential stress or von Mises stress) and strength is still matter of controversy. Gaining an understanding of the mechanical properties of the AAA tissue therefore is of clinical significance. Due to the difficult to reliably predict abdominal aortic aneurysm expansion and rupture in individuals several clinical trials have been performed [25, 72]. At the same time, from the computational point of view, literature systematically reports the evidence to support the role of patient-specific biomechanical profiles in the management of patients with AAA both from imaging and FE approach [1, 13, 81]. In order to accurately predict the risk of rupture of AAA, is necessary to predict the AAA wall strength distribution and the material properties non-invasively. With regard to our work, our specific FE simulations (both deterministic and probabilistic), reveal the importance to define a more realistic geometrical shape by including also wall thickness regional variation. Several previous studies were devoted to the definition of the geometrical parameters that mainly influence the wall stress (Vorp et al. [83] and more recently Rodríguez et al. [62] found that wall stress is substantially increased by an asymmetric bulge in AAAs, just to cite but a few), but, to the best of our knowledge, this is the first structural study in which also the wall thickness is considered as variable. Figure 15 depicts results from two deterministic simulations extracted by the multivariate analysis: aneurysm with a large diameter and constant wall thickness (a) and FE model small diameter and a wall thickness reduction of 50% in the ventral area. The stress contour plot points out how the wall thickness reduction influence the maximum stress value and its localization.

To conclude, there is, therefore, a pressing need to include patient specific regional variations to identify regions within AAAs that have the highest ratio of stress to strength. Future studies on patient-specific geometries of AAAs should consider the actual wall thickness. Moreover, the understanding the mechanical properties of the AAA wall will enhance our ability to design implants that can stay in place and/or protect the aneurysm wall from blood pressure.

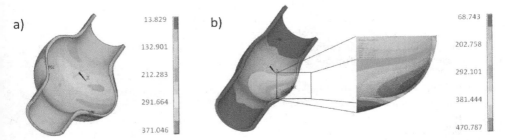

Figure 15. Stress contour plot of aneurysm with a large diameter and constant wall thickness (a) and a FE model small diameter and a wall thickness reduction of 50% in the ventral area.

Author details

Simona Celi
Institute of Clinical Physiology National Research Council IFC-CNR, Massa
Fondazione Toscana CNR "G. Monasterio", Heart Hospital, Massa, Italy

Sergio Berti
Fondazione Toscana CNR "G. Monasterio", Heart Hospital, Massa, Italy

6. References

[1] Abbas, A., Attia, R., Smith, A. & M.Waltham [2011]. Can we predict abdominal aortic aneurysm (aaa) progression and rupture by non-invasive imaging?-a systematic review, *International Journal of Clinical Medicine* 2: 484–499.

[2] Alexander, J. J. [2004]. The pathobiology of aortic aneurysms, *Journal of Surgical Research* 117: 163–175.

[3] Ang, A. S. & Tang, W. H. [1984]. *Probabilistic concepts in engineering planning and design, Decision, risk and reliability*, John Wiley & Sons Inc.

[4] Baek, S., Gleason, R., Rajagopal, K. & Humphrey, J. [2007]. Theory of small on large: Potential utility in computations of fluidŨsolid interactions in arteries, *Computer Methods in Applied Mechanics and Engineering* 196: 3070–3078.

[5] Basciano, C. A. & Kleinstreuer, C. [2009]. Invariant-based anisotropic constitutive models of the healthy and aneurysmal abdominal aortic wall, *Journal of Biomechanical Engineering* 131(2): 021009 (11 pages).

[6] Boehler, J. P. [1987]. *Introduction to the Invariant Formulation of Anisotropic Constitutive Equations*, Springer-Verlag, Wien„ chapter Applications of Tensor Functions in Solid Mechanics, CISM Courses and Lectures No., 292, pp. 13–30.

[7] Borghi, A., Wood, N., Mohiaddin, R. & Xu, X. [2006]. 3d geometric reconstruction of thoracic aortic aneurysms, *BioMedical Engineering OnLine* 5(59): 1–13.

[8] Celi, S. [2012]. Numerical and experimental simulations of surgical procedures, *PhD Thesis*, University of Pisa.

[9] Celi, S. & Berti, S. [2012]. FE simulations on the effect of regional variations of material properties and wall thickness on AAA, *GNB congress*, ISBN: 978 88 555 3182-5.

[10] Celi, S., Berti, S., Mariani, M., Di Puccio, F. & Forte, P. [2010]. Investigation on the effect of the wall thickness in rupture risk estimation of aaa by a probabilistic finite element approach, *European Heart Journal* 31 (Supp)(1): 284.

[11] Celi, S., Di Puccio, F. & Forte, P. [2011]. Advances in finite element simulations of elastosonography for breast lesion detection, *Journal of Biomechanical Engineering* 133: 081006–13.

[12] Choi, H. S. & Vito, R. P. [1990]. Two-dimensional stress-strain relationship for canine pericardium, *Journal of Biomechanical Engineering* 112(2): 153–159.

[13] Choke, E., Cockerill, G., Wilson, W., Sayed, S., Dawson, J., Loftus, I. & Thompson, M. [2005]. A review of biological factors implicated in abdominal aortic aneurysm rupture, *European Journal of Vascular and Endovascular Surgery* 30(3): 227–244.

[14] Chuong, C. J. & Fung, Y. C. [1983]. Three-dimensional stress distribution in arteries, *Journal of Biomechanical Engineering* 105(3): 268–274.

[15] Cox, R. [1978]. Regional variation of series elasticity in canine arterial smooth muscles., *American Journal of Physiology* 234(5): H542–51.

[16] Darling, R., Messina, C., Brewster, D. & Ottinger, L. [1977]. Autopsy study of unoperated abdominal aortic aneurysms, *Circulation* 56: 161–164.

[17] Di Achille, P., Celi, S., Di Puccio, F. & Forte, P. [2011]. Anisotropic aaa: computational comparison between four and two fiber family material models, *Journal of Biomechanics* 44(13): 2418–26.

[18] Di Martino, E., Bohra, A., Geest, J. V., Gupta, N. & Vorp, M. M. D. [2006]. Biomechanical properties of ruptured versus electively repaired abdominal aortic aneurysm wall tissue, *Journal of Vascular Surgery* 43(3): 570–576.

[19] Di Puccio, F., Celi, S. & Forte, P. [2012]. Review of experimental investigations on compressibility of arteries and the introduction of a new apparatus, *Experimental Mechanics* 52(7): 1–8, DOI: 10.1007/s11340-012-9614-4.

[20] Dingemans, K., Teeling, P., Lagendijk, J. & Becker, A. [2000]. Extracellular matrix of the human aortic media: an ultrastructural histochemical and immunohistochemical study of the adult aortic media, *The Anatomical Record* 258(1): 1–14.

[21] Dobrin, P. [1989]. Pathophysiology and pathogenesis of aortic aneurysms. current concepts, *Surgical Clinics of North America Journal* 69(4): 687–703.

[22] Ferruzzi, J., Vorp, D. A. & Humphrey, J. D. [2011]. On constitutive descriptors of the biaxial mechanical behaviour of human abdominal aorta and aneurysms, *Journal of the Royal Society Interface* 8: 435–450.

[23] Fillinger, M. F., Marra, S. P., Raghavan, M. L. & Kennedy, F. E. [2003]. Prediction of rupture risk in abdominal aortic aneurysm during observation: wall stress versus diameter, *Journal of Vascular Surgery* 37: 724–732.

[24] Fillinger, M. F., Raghavan, M. L., Marra, S. P., C., J. L. & Kennedy, F. E. [2002]. In vivo analysis of mechanical wall stress and abdominal aortic aneurysm rupture risk, *Journal of Vascular Surgery* 36(3): 589–597.

[25] Fleming, C., Whitlock, E. P., Beil, T. L. & Lederle, F. A. [2005]. Screening for abdominal aortic aneurysm: A best-evidence systematic review for the u.s. preventive services task force, *Annals of Internal Medicine* 142(3): 203–211.

[26] Fung, Y. C., Fronek, K. & Patitucci, P. [1979]. Pseudoelasticity of arteries and the choice of its mathematical expression, *American Journal of Physiology* 237(5): AH620–31.

[27] Ganten, M. K., Krautter, U., von Tengg-Kobligk, H., H., D. B., Schumacher, Stiller, W., Delorme, S., Kauczor, H., Kauffmann, G. & Bock, M. [2008]. Quantification of aortic

distensibility in abdominal aortic aneurysm using ecg-gated multi-detector computed tomography, *Vascular-Interventional* 18(5): 966–73.

[28] Gasser, T. C. [2011]. An irreversible constitutive model for fibrouss of tbiological tissue: a 3d microfiber approach with demonstrative application to abdominal aorticaneurysms, *Acta Biomaterialia* 7(6): 2457–2466.

[29] Gasser, T. C., Auer, M., Labruto, F., Roy, J. & Swedenborg, J. [2009]. Using finite element analysis to assess rupture risk in abdominal aortic aneurysms including the effect of the intraluminal thrombus., *Journal of Vascular Surgery* 49(5): S29.

[30] Greenwald, S. E. [2007]. Ageing of the conduit arteries, *Journal of Pathology* 211: 157–172.

[31] Haskett, D., Johnson, G., Zhou, A., Utzinger, U. & Vande Geest, J. [2010]. Microstructural and biomechanical alterations of the human aorta as a function of age and location, *Biomechanics and Modeling in Mechanobiology* 9: 725–736. 10.1007/s10237-010-0209-7.

[32] He, C. M. & Roach, M. [1994]. The composition and mechanical properties of abdominal aortic aneurysms, *Journal of Vascular Surgery* 20(1): 6–13.

[33] Holzapfel, G. A. [2000]. *Holzapfel, G. A., 2000, Nonlinear Solid Mechanics: A Continuum Approach for Engineering, Wiley, England*, Wiley, England.

[34] Holzapfel, G. A., Gasser, T. C. & Ogden, R. W. [2000]. A new constitutive framework for arterial wall mechanics and a comparative study of material models, *Journal of Elasticity* 61: 1–48.

[35] Holzapfel, G. A., Gasser, T. C. & Stadler, M. [2002]. A structural model for the viscoelastic behavior of arterial walls: continuum formulation and finite element analysis, *European Journal of Mechanic–A/Solids* 21(3): 441–463.

[36] Humphrey, J. D. [1995]. Mechanics of the arterial wall: review and directions, *Critical reviewsinbiomedicalengineering* 23(1Ǔ2): 1–162.

[37] Humphrey, J. D. [2008]. Vascular adaptation and mechanical homeostasis at tissue, cellular, and sub-cellular levels, *Cell Biochem. Biophys.* 50: 53–78.

[38] Humphrey, J. D. & Rajagopal, K. R. [2002]. A constrained mixture model for growth and remodeling of soft tissues, *Mathematical Models and Methods in Applied Sciences* 12: 407–430.

[39] Humphrey, J. D. & Rajagopal, K. R. [2003]. A constrained mixture model for arterial adaptations to a sustained step change in blood flow, *Biomech Model Mechanobiol* 2(2): 109–26.

[40] Humphrey, J. D. & Yin, F. C. [1987]. A new constitutive formulation for characterizing the mechanical behavior of soft tissues, *Biophysical Journal* 52(4): 563–570.

[41] Kuhl, E. & Holzapfel, G. A. [2007]. A continuum model for remodeling in living structures, *Journal of Materials Science* 42: 8811–8823.

[42] Li, Z.-Y., Sadat, U., U-King-Im, J., Tang, T. Y., Bowden, D. J., Hayes, P. D. & Gillard, J. H. [2010]. Association between aneurysm shoulder stress and abdominal aortic aneurysm expansion. a longitudinal follow-up study, *Circulation* 122: 1815–1822.

[43] Länne, T., Sonesson, B., Bergqvist, D., Bengtsson, H. & Gustafsson, D. [1992]. Diameter and compliance in the male human abdominal aorta: influence of age and aortic aneurysm, *European Journal of Vascular Surgery* 6(2): 178–184.

[44] MacSweeney, S. T., Young, G., Greenhalgh, R. M. & Powell, J. T. [1992]. Mechanical properties of the aneurysmal aorta, *British Journal of Surgery* 79(12): 1281–4.

[45] Maier, A., Gee, M. W., Reeps, C., Eckstein, H. H. & Wall, W. A. [2010]. Impact of calcifications on patient-specific wall stress analysis of abdominal aortic aneurysms., *Biomech. Model. Mechanobiol.* 9(5): 511–21.

[46] McKay, M. D., Beckman, R. J. & Conover, W. J. [1979]. A comparison of three methods for selecting values of input variables in the analysis of output from a computer code, *Technometrics* 42: 55–61.

[47] Molacek, J., Baxa, J., Houdek, K., Treska, V. & Ferda, J. [2011]. Assessment of abdominal aortic aneurysm wall distensibility with electrocardiography-gated computed tomography, *Annals of Vascular Surgery* 25(8): 1036–1042.

[48] Murphy, S. L., Xu, J. & Kochanek, K. D. [2012]. Deaths: Preliminary data for 2010, *National Vital Statistics System* 60(4): 1–68.

[49] Nichols, W. W. & O'Rourke, M. [1997]. *Mcdonald's Blood Flow in Arteries: Theoretical, Experimental and Clinical Principles (4th ed.)*, Hodder Arnold Publication.

[50] Ogden, R. W. [2009]. Anisotropy and nonlinear elasticity in arterial wall mechanics, *in* G. A. Holzapfel, R. W. Ogden, F. Pfeiffer, F. G. Rammerstorfer, J. Salençon, B. Schrefler & P. Serafini (eds), *Biomechanical Modelling at the Molecular, Cellular and Tissue Levels*, Vol. 508 of *CISM Courses and Lectures*, Springer Vienna, pp. 179–258.

[51] O'Rourke, M. F. & Hashimoto, J. [2007]. Mechanical factors in arterial aging: A clinical perspective, *Journal of the American College of Cardiology* 50: 1–13.

[52] Polzer, S., Gasser, T., Swedenborg, J. & Bursa, J. [2011]. The impact of intraluminal thrombus failure on the mechanical stress in the wall of abdominal aortic aneurysms, *European Journal of Vascular and Endovascular Surgery* 41(4): 467–473.

[53] Raghavan, M. L. & da Silva, E. S. [2011]. *Studies in Mechanobiology, Tissue Engineering and Biomaterials*, Springer, chapter Mechanical Properties of AAA Tissue, pp. 139–162.

[54] Raghavan, M. L., Kratzberg, J., de Tolosa, E. M. C., Hanaoka, M. M., Walker, P. & da Silva, E. S. [2006]. Regional distribution of wall thickness and failure properties of human abdominal aortic aneurysm, *Journal of Biomechanics* 39: 3010–3016.

[55] Raghavan, M. L., Vorp, D. A., Federle, M. P., Makaroun, M. S. & Webster, M. W. [2000]. Wall stress distribution on three-dimensionally reconstructed models of human abdominal aortic aneurysm, *Journal of Vascular Surgery* 31: 760–769.

[56] Raghavan, M. & Vorp, D. [2000]. Toward a biomechanical tool to evaluate rupture potential of abdominal aortic aneurysm: identification of a finite strain constitutive model and evaluation of its applicability, *Journal of Biomechanics* 33(4): 475–82.

[57] Raghavan, M., Webster, M. & Vorp, D. [1996]. Ex vivo biomechanical behavior of abdominal aortic aneurysm: assessment using a new mathematical model, *Ann. Biomed. Eng* 24(5): 573–582.

[58] Reh, S., Beley, J.-D., Mukherjee, S. & Khor, E. H. [2006]. Probabilistic finite element analysis using ansys, *Structural Safety* 28: 17–43.

[59] Rissland, P., Alemu, Y., Einav, S., Ricotta, J. & Bluestein, D. . [2009]. Abdominal aortic aneurysm risk of rupture: patientspecific fsi simulations using anisotropic model, *Journal of Biomechanical Engineering* 131(3): 031001.

[60] Rizzo, R. J., McCarthy, W. J., Dixit, S. N., Lilly, M. P., Shively, V. P., Flinn, W. R. & Yao, J. S. T. [1989]. Collagen types and matrix protein content in human abdominal aortic aneurysms, *Journal of Vascular Surgery* 10: 365–373.

[61] Roach, M. R. & Burton, A. C. [1957]. The reason for the shape of the distensibility curves of arteries, *Canadian Journal of Biochemistry and Physiology* 35(8): 681–690.

[62] Rodríguez, J. F., Ruiz, C., Doblaré, M. & Holzapfel, G. A. [2008]. Mechanical stresses in abdominal aortic aneurysms: influence of diameter, asymmetry, and material anisotropy, *Journal of Biomechanical Engineering* 130(2): 021023.

[63] Rodríguez, J., Martufi, G., Doblaré, M. & Finol, E. [2009]. The effect of material model formulation in the stress analysis of abdominal aortic aneurysms, *Annals of Biomedical Engineering* 37: 2218–2221.

[64] Sacks, M. [2000]. Biaxial mechanical evaluation of planar biological materials, *Journal of Elasticity* 61($\aleph_0$): 199–246.

[65] Sakalihasan, N., Limet, R. & Defawe, O. [2005]. Abdominal aortic aneurysm, *Lancet* 365(9470): 1577–1589.

[66] Schriefl, A. J., Zeindlinger, G., Pierce, D. M., Regitnig, P. & Holzapfel, G. A. [2011]. Determination of the layer-specific distributed collagen fibre orientations in human thoracic and abdominal aortas and common iliac arteries, *Journal of The Royal Society Interface* doi:10.1098/rsif.2011.0727: on line.

[67] Scotti, C. M., Jimenez, J., Muluk, S. C. & Finol, E. A. [2008]. Wall stress and flow dynamics in abdominal aortic aneurysms: finite element analysis vs. fluid-structure interaction, *Computer Methods in Biomechanics and Biomedical Engineering* 11: 301–322.

[68] Speelman, L. A., Bohra, A., Bosboom, E. M. H., Schurink, G. W. H., van de Vosse, F. N., Makaroun, M. S. & Vorp, D. A. [2007]. Effects of wall calcifications in patient-specific wall stress analyses of abdominal aortic aneurysms., *Journal of Biomechanical Engineering* 129(1): 105–109.

[69] Spencer, A. J. M. [1984]. *Continuum Theory of the Mechanics of Fibre-Reinforced Composites*, Springer-Verlag, chapter Continuum Theory of the Mechanics of Fibre-Reinforced Composites, CISM Courses and Lectures No. 282, pp. 1–32.

[70] Thubrikar, M., Labrosse, M., Robicsek, F., Al-Soudi, J. & Fowler, B. [2001]. Mechanical properties of abdominal aortic aneurysm wall, *Journal of Medical Engineering & Technology* 25(4): 133–42.

[71] United Kingdom EVAR Trial Investigators, Greenhalgh, R., Brown, L., Powell, J., Thompson, S., Epstein, D. & Sculpher, M. [2010]. Endovascular versus open repair of abdominal aortic aneurysm, *New England Journal of Medicine* 362: 1863–1871.

[72] U.S. Preventive Services Task Force [2005]. Screening for abdominal aortic aneurysm: Recommendation statement, *Annals of Internal Medicine* 142(3): 198–202.

[73] Vaishnav, R. N., Young, J. T., Janicki, J. S. & Patel, J. S. [1972]. Non linear anisotropic elastic properties of the canine aorta, *Biophysical Journal* 12(8): 1008–1027.

[74] Valenta, J. [1993]. *Clinical Aspects of Biomedicine*, Elsevier.

[75] van St Veer, M., Buth, J., Merkx, M., Tonino, P., van den Bosch, H., Pijls, N. & van de Vosse, F. [2008]. Biomechanical properties of abdominal aortic aneurysms assessed by simultaneously measured pressure and volume changes in humans, *Journal of Vascular Surgery* 48(6): 1401–1407.

[76] Vande Geest, J. P., Sacks, M. S. & Vorp, D. A. [2004]. Age dependency of the biaxial biomechanical behavior of human abdominal aorta, *Journal of Biomechanical Engineering* 12: 815–822.

[77] Vande Geest, J. P., Sacks, M. S. & Vorp, D. A. [2006]. The effects of aneurysm on the biaxial mechanical behavior of human abdominal aorta, *Journal of Biomechanics* 39: 1324–1334.

[78] Vande Geest, J. P., Wang, D. H. J., Wisniewski, S. R., Makaroun, M. S. & Vorp, D. A. [2006]. Towards a noninvasive method for determination of patient-specific wall strength distribution in abdominal aortic aneurysms, *Ann. Biomed. Eng.* 34(7): 1098–106.

[79] Venkatasubramaniam, A., Fagan, M., Mehta, T., Mylankal, K., Ray, B., Kuhan, G., Chetter, I. & McCollum, P. [2004]. A comparative study of aortic wall stress using finite element

analysis for ruptured and non- ruptured abdominal aortic aneurysms, *European Journal of Vascular Surgery* 28: 168–176.

[80] Vito, R. P. & Dixon, S. A. [2003]. Blood vessel constitutive models: 1995Ű2002, *Annu. Rev. Biomed. Eng.* 5(No. 0): 413–439.

[81] Vorp, D. A. [2007]. Biomechanics of abdominal aortic aneurysm, *Journal of Biomechanics* 40: 1887–1902.

[82] Vorp, D. A., Raghavan, M. L., Muluk, S. C., Makaroun, M. S., Steed, D. L., Shapiro, R. & Webster, M. W. [1996]. Wall strength and stiffness of aneurysmal and nonaneurysmal abdominal aorta, *Annals of the New York Academy of Sciences* 800(1): 274–276.

[83] Vorp, D. A., Raghavan, M. L. & Webster, M. W. [1998]. Mechanical wall stress in abdominal aortic aneurysm: influence of diameter and asymmetry, *Journal of Vascular Surgery* 27: 632–639.

[84] Vorp, D., Lee, P., Wang, D., Makaroun, M., Nemoto, E., Ogawa, S. & MW., M. W. [2001]. Association of intraluminal thrombus in abdominal aortic aneurysm with local hypoxia and wall weakening, *Journal of Vascular Surgery* 34: 291–9.

[85] Wang, D. H. J., Makaroun, M. S., Webster, M. W. & Vorp, D. A. [2002]. Effect of intraluminal thrombus on wall stress in patient-specific models of abdominal aortic aneurysm, *Journal of Vascular Surgery* 36: 598–604.

[86] Wicker, B. K., Hutchens, H. P., Wu, Q., Yeh, A. T. & Humphrey, J. D. [2008]. Normal basilar artery structure and biaxial mechanical behaviour, *Computer Methods in Biomechanics and Biomedical Engineering* 11: 539–551.

[87] Zeinali-Davarani, S., Choi, J. & Baek, S. [2009]. On parameter estimation for biaxial mechanical behavior of arteries, *Journal of Biomechanics* 42: 524–530.

Chapter 2

Main Models of Experimental Saccular Aneurysm in Animals

Ivanilson Alves de Oliveira

Additional information is available at the end of the chapter

1. Introduction

Intracranial saccular aneurysms are lesions of the arteries, the etiology of which remains controversial. Some evidence indicates that intracranial saccular aneurysms arise from a congenital deficiency of the smooth muscle of the arterial wall and local hemodynamic disorders particularly in areas of arterial bifurcation [1], [2]. These aneurysms are less commonly due to trauma, tumors, infections, use of drugs, and conditions associated with high arterial flow {e.g., arteriovenous malformations (AVM)} and connective tissue diseases [3-11]. Saccular aneurysms might be single or multiple and are mostly located in the Circle of Willis. These aneurysms are the most frequent cause of spontaneous subarachnoid hemorrhage (SAH) and primarily affect females. Patients become symptomatic after rupture, which usually occurs between ages 40 to 60 years old[12]. Because rupture is associated with high morbidity and mortality rates, appropriate treatment must be performed as soon as possible. The aim of the treatment is to exclude the aneurysm from the circulation to avoid further bleeding, while preserving the parent artery [13, 14]. Currently, two techniques are available for the treatment of saccular aneurysms: 1) microsurgery (developed by Yasargil), which is based on the placement of a metallic clip in the aneurysm neck [15], and 2) endovascular coiling (developed by Guglielmi), which is based on the introduction of platinum microcoils inside the aneurysms that induce thrombosis and thus isolate aneurysms from the circulation[16]. The continuous development of this latter technique has reduced the morbidity and mortality of the treatment of brain aneurysms [17]; however, improvement of models of experimental saccular aneurysms is needed to develop novel embolization techniques and to test new materials.

2. Selection of the animal species

2.1. Concept of experimental animal

The terms "laboratory animal" or "experimental animal" are somewhat inappropriate because in theory, any animal can be used in laboratory experiments. Nevertheless, both terms are frequently used in scientific literature to refer to animals exhibiting (natural or induced) diseases in which the mechanisms are similar to human diseases.

2.2. Types of experimental models with animals

Experimental models with animals are classified as: 1) induced, 2) spontaneous, 3) negative and 4) orphan[18]. In the induced animal models, the investigated condition is induced experimentally, which can be highly advantageous because these models allow for free selection of the animal species, for example, intake of beta-aminopropionitrile combined with arterial hypertension induces intracranial aneurysm formation in rats [19]. Induced animal models are very important in the development of novel surgical procedures, to assess the viability of procedures and their physiological consequences, and in therapeutic assays, for instance, the surgical creation of aneurysms on the lateral wall of the common carotid artery of dogs [20] and pigs [21]. In spontaneous models, the investigated disease occurs naturally, such as with prostatic hypertrophy in dogs and some diseases in animals with genetic mutations. The spontaneous occurrence of intracranial saccular aneurysms in animals is rare. Negative models involve a particular disease that does not develop in a particular species and, thus, these models are ideal to study mechanisms of resistance or a lack of reactivity to a given stimulus. For example, rabbits do not develop gonorrhea and vultures do no exhibit neoplasms. In orphan models, a disease (or condition) that occurs naturally in non-human species is "adopted" when a similar human disease is identified at a later time (e.g., bovine spongiform encephalopathy, which is also known as mad cow disease) [18].

2.3. Principles for animal selection

Experimental animals should only be used when there are limitations to the research with humans. In therapeutic assays, the use of animals is mandatory and constitutes an essential phase of the preclinical testing of embolization devices or materials. In general, small animals are the most frequently used for research purposes; mice, rats, rabbits, and guinea pigs correspond to 90% of scientific studies [22]. Larger animals such as dogs [20], pigs [21], or monkeys [23] are also used for research purposes, albeit less frequently. Such diversity of species that exhibit different characteristics makes it difficult to select a particular species for experimental aneurysm production. Although there are no specific guidelines on how to perform such a selection, three general principles must be considered: 1) the type of animal that will be used, 2) the type of aneurysm one seeks to simulate, and 3) the aims of the study.

Regarding the animal type, researchers should be thoroughly aware of its biological characteristics, behavior, vascular anatomy, and phylogenetic similarity with humans.

Among the biological characteristics, the size and metabolism of the animals exert a direct influence on the selection. Large animals are more difficult to handle and require more complex infrastructure (lodging, feeding, care, anesthesia, and specialized human resources), which increases the cost of research. In addition, size also influences the number of animals used in experiments. Thus, for ethical reasons, studies that use large animals such as dogs and monkeys restrict their number to the bare minimum needed to ensure the validity of the results. A reduced number of animals influences the statistical methods applied to the analysis, because small samples can reduce the statistical power of tests and lead researchers to infer inaccurate conclusions. In addition, the calculation of the minimum number of animals is difficult because unpredictable losses can also occur as a function of the initial training and pilot study.

With regard to metabolism, different animal species also exhibit different patterns of metabolic rate; for instance, the metabolism of rodents is often faster than that of humans. This metabolic power (also known as metabolic body weight) interferes with the effects of drugs on the organism, as well as with its processing, distribution across organic fluids and tissues, and modes of excretion. Thus, the calculation of experimental doses should be performed according to the metabolic weight rather than the absolute body weight of the animals. In surgical studies, different metabolic rates (influenced by factors such as age, gender, diet, and circadian rhythm) interfere with wound healing and regeneration of tissues and organs, thus encouraging researchers to learn the principles of veterinary anesthesia that correspond to the involved animals, the characteristics of the drugs that will be used, and more specifically, the potential interference of medications with the parameters analyzed in the study[18].

In addition to the biological characteristics, researchers must also be familiar with the intracranial and cervical arterial anatomy of each animal species, and the histology, diameters, flow patterns, and anastomoses of the vessels, because these are essential factors in the selection of the aneurysm construction technique.

The phylogenetic similarity between animals and humans is also important in species selection, but it does not suggest that the extrapolation of the results to humans will be reliable. For example, human immunodeficiency virus (HIV) does not induce immunodeficiency in monkeys, and thus, does not represent the ideal animal model to study acquired immunodeficiency syndrome (AIDS). Transgenic animals have been increasingly used in research studies; however, caution is needed because such animals might exhibit unknown disorders that may interfere with the extrapolation of the results to humans[18].

Once the animal model has been selected, the experiment performed, and the data selected, the stage of explaining the phenomena by means of induction begins. This process consists of verifying a particular fact and its adequation to a known general law. This mode of reasoning has inherent odds of error; thus, one must be cautious in the extrapolation of the results of experiments performed with non-human species to humans. In other words, compounds that might be noxious to a given non-human species might be innocuous or even beneficial to humans. For example, penicillin is lethal for guinea pigs, but is well tolerated and even beneficial for humans. In addition, aspirin is teratogenic in cats, dogs, rats, guinea pigs, mice, and monkeys, but it is innocuous in pregnant women. Thalidomide is teratogenic in human beings and monkeys, but innocuous in rats and other species. Therefore, phylogenetic proximity is not a fully reliable measure of similarity between the physiological phenomena of animals and humans [18].

To reduce the odds of selecting an inappropriate animal model for a given experiment, the *multispecies approach* is recommended. At least two different species including non-rodents must be used in studies employing drugs, whereas the use of more than one animal species is rare in studies of surgical techniques. Accordingly, some animal species have become traditional standard models for specific surgical procedures. However, surgical studies focusing on the physiological features of a disease require more than one animal species, which despite its usefulness, does not ensure the absolute reliability of the extrapolation of the results from animals to humans [18].

Regarding the aneurysm model, a comprehensive awareness of the available models is required, in addition to their construction techniques, advantages and disadvantages, and more specifically, which features of human aneurysms one seeks to simulate, that is, their histological, geometric, physiopathological, and hemodynamic characteristics (e.g., ruptured or not, small, medium-sized, large or giant, with or without thrombus, on the lateral wall or at a bifurcation, high or low hemodynamic tension, etc.).

Finally, the aims of the study are essential in the selection of the animal species and the techniques that will be used in aneurysm construction, e.g., verification of the physiopathological mechanisms, therapeutic assays, creation of novel surgical/endovascular techniques, or training of doctors in these therapeutic modalities. Regarding the latter issue, medical training using animals is justified as training on humans exposes patients to medical error. Thus, practical training using animal models is indispensable for medical education because it contributes to the development of psychomotor skills and enables physicians to safely perform invasive techniques.

2.4. Main animal species used in the construction of experimental saccular aneurysms

Despite all of the considerations above, the selection of the ideal animal species for studies on experimental saccular aneurysms is not yet well established. As spontaneous intracranial aneurysms rarely occur in animals, most studies employ induced models, which have the advantage of allowing for the free selection of species. Animals such as rats[19], rabbits[24], dogs[20], pigs[21], and monkeys[23] have been used in studies on physiopathology [25, 26], hemodynamics[27-31], and the training of surgical[32, 33] and endovascular techniques, in addition to the testing of embolization devices and new materials[21, 34-38]. In studies aimed at developing surgical/endovascular techniques, it is rare that more than one animal species is used in the same experimental model; therefore, there are no systematic comparative studies seeking to define which is the ideal animal species for the experimental production of intracranial saccular aneurysms. Nevertheless, in recent years, rabbits (*Oryctolagus cuniculus*) have been preferred for these studies because their coagulation system is very similar to that of humans. Rabbits are easy to handle, and the diameters of their extracranial carotid arteries are very similar to those of humans [39-44].

2.5. Cervicocerebral vascular anatomy of rabbits

Regarding the vascular anatomy of rabbits, knowledge of the cervicocerebral vessels and their connections is essential in the construction of experimental saccular aneurysms. Below, we present a summary of the cervical and intracranial vascular anatomy of rabbits together with their main anastomoses.

The innominate artery (3.5 mm in diameter) is the first branch of the aortic arch, and after running 6 mm, it divides into the right subclavian (2 mm in diameter) and right common carotid (2 mm of diameter) arteries. The left common carotid artery (2 mm in diameter) begins immediately next to or together with the innominate artery. The left subclavian artery (2 mm in diameter) is the last branch of the aortic arch, and it originates from the left vertebral (1 mm in diameter) and superficial cervical (1 mm in diameter) arteries[45]. In the second most frequent distribution type, the aortic arch can only be divided into three branches: the innominate, left common carotid, and left subclavian arteries. Lesser variations might also occur; for instance, the supreme intercostal and left vertebral arteries might originate directly from the aortic arch. The superior thyroid artery usually originates from the common carotid arteries; however, it emerges approximately between the 3rd and 6th tracheal rings and runs towards the thyroid gland, in some cases of only one common carotid artery[46]. Upon arriving at the isthmus, the superior thyroid artery divides into two branches: one ascending (cricothyroid branch) and the other descending (which runs inferiorly between the trachea and the esophagus). The bronchial branches stem from the right supreme intercostal and left common carotid arteries and lead to the tracheoesophageal branches, which run upwards between the trachea and the esophagus and anastomose with the descending branches of the superior thyroid artery[47] (figure 1). These branches rarely exhibit variations, and when they do occur, these variations are more common on the left side[48].

The common carotid artery (CCA) leads to only one branch, namely the thyroid artery, and immediately above it, the CCA divides into the internal and external carotid arteries. The main branches of the external carotid artery (ECA) are the occipital, lingual, external maxillary (facial), and anterior and posterior auricular arteries. Both the auricular and external maxillary arteries emerge separately or from a common trunk. At the level of the zygomatic arch, the ECA divides into the superficial temporal and transverse facial arteries and continues its course up to the pterygoid canal, where it divides into small branches to the posterior side of the orbit and originates the external ophthalmic artery, which in turn forms the lacrimal and frontal branches, and subsequently, the anastomose with the internal ophthalmic artery. The main branch of the internal maxillary artery is the middle meningeal artery. The intracranial internal carotid artery (ICA) divides into the ophthalmic arteries, cranial, and caudal branches. The cranial branch runs forward towards the uncus, where it divides into the anterior choroidal artery and middle cerebral artery (MCA) trunk, and then continues up to the chiasm, where it unites with the contralateral cranial branch to form a common anterior cerebral artery trunk that separates again at the level of the corpus callosum. The common anterior trunk originates from the lateral artery of the olfactory bulb, which leads to the ethmoidal branches of the cribiform plate. The MCA runs along the lateral cerebral sulcus and divides into the posterior ophthalmic artery, large posterior branch, and large anterior and middle branches, in addition to the small olfactory bulb branches. The caudal branch of the ICA supplies most of the blood flow of the basilar artery (BA) and leads to the following branches: posterior communicating artery, small medial geniculate body branches, large anterior quadrigeminal body, small branches of the posterior side of the uncus, and the posterior segment of the corpus callosum. The cerebellar artery might originate from the ending of the ICA or the BA and connects to several branches of the brainstem. The BA is formed by the fusion of the arteries of the first spinal nerves and divides (on the ventral surface of the trapezoid body) into two vessels that reunite at the upper margin of the pons. In addition, the BA gives small lateral branches, the cerebellar artery and the perforating branches. The arteries of the first spinal nerve then reunite at a lower level and form the ventral spinal artery[49].

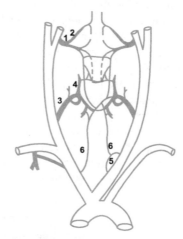

Figure 1. Graphic representation of the visceral vascularization of the neck of rabbits. 1- superior laryngeal artery, 2- superior branches, 3- superior thyroid artery, 4- cricothyroid branch, 5- bronchial branch and 6- tracheoesophageal branch. Modified from Bugge, 1967[2].

Regarding the system of intracranial anastomoses in rabbits, the collateral circulation is very different from that of dogs. The internal maxillary artery originates from the orbital branches, which end at the ophthalmic branch and represents an insufficient anastomotic pathway. The anastomotic branches between the orbital and internal carotid arteries are too small or are absent. A small branch links together the ICA and BA before they unite at the circle. Finally, when an occlusion of the common carotid artery occurs, the supply of blood is provided by the contralateral ICA (**figure 2**)[3].

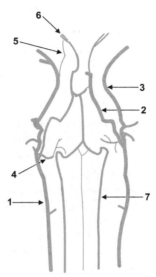

Figure 2. Graphic representation of the intracranial anastomosis system of rabbits. 1- common carotid artery, 2- internal carotid artery, 3- external carotid artery, 4- occipital artery, 5- orbital artery, 6 – internal ophthalmic artery and 7- vertebral artery. Modified from Chungcharoen, 1954[50].

3. Selection of an experimental saccular aneurysm model

3.1. Concept of experimental saccular aneurysm

Experimental saccular aneurysms are induced aneurysms intended to reproduce the histological, geometric, and hemodynamic characteristics of human intracranial aneurysms.

3.2. Characteristics of an ideal model of experimental saccular aneurysm

With the rise of endovascular treatment of human intracranial aneurysms – by means of embolization using platinum microcoils[16] – experimental models of saccular aneurysm are encouraged to adapt to this novel therapeutic modality by meeting the following criteria: 1) demonstration of long-term permeability in untreated control species, 2) development in animal species with a coagulation system similar to that of humans, 3) simulation of the morphology of arterial bifurcation, terminal artery, or other aneurysmal types that expose the aneurysm neck to high hemodynamic tension, 4) development in vessels with a similar size to human intracranial vessels, 5) development without the need of local surgery to minimize the repair/wound healing response, which might confound the results of the experiment with the natural increase of the biological activity characteristic of several embolization materials such as: coils, fluid agents, etc., and 6) simulation of the limitations met by embolization of human aneurysms using such materials[39].

3.3. Main models of experimental saccular aneurysm

German and Black (1954) were the first researchers to produce experimental aneurysms using a surgical construction of saccular aneurysms on the common carotid artery of dogs. Such aneurysms mimicked the ones occurring on the lateral wall and were frequently used in hemodynamic studies; however, they produced fibrosis at the suture site, which was a disadvantage[20]. Since then, surgical models have evolved with the culmination of the swine model (1994), consisting of a graft of the venous pouch onto the common carotid artery (CCA) of pigs. This method produces lateral wall aneurysms, but includes disadvantages such as venous histology, induction of intense fibrosis at the suture site, and low hemodynamic tension[16].

In addition to the surgical method, chemical induction might also be used in the construction of saccular aneurysms. The main proponent of this technique was Hashimoto (1970), who induced arterial wall weakening in rats by ingestion of 3-beta-aminopropionitrile, a toxic agent extracted from the seeds of the sweat pea (*Latyrus odoratus*), which destroys the elastic fibers and collagen of the arteries of rats[19]. In addition, Hashimoto ligated one of the common carotid arteries and induced arterial hypertension in rats (via nephrectomy, intake of saline solution, and high doses of corticosteroids) to cause greater hemodynamic tension on the weakened arterial wall[30]. This technique was the first to produce successful intracranial saccular aneurysms at the bifurcations of the cerebral arterial circle. Nonetheless, the aneurysms were too small and were not useful for the development of surgical techniques nor for the study of intra-aneurysmal hemodynamic alterations[26, 29].

3.3.1. Surgical models

The technique used in the surgical construction of experimental aneurysm is based on grafting a venous pouch (usually taken from the external jugular vein) onto the common carotid artery. The main advantage of this approach is that the constructed aneurysms exhibit hemodynamic features that are very similar to those of humans. the disadvantages of constructed aneurysms include their venous histology and resistance to rupture.

With regard to the construction site, the graft might be placed on the lateral wall or at bifurcations. There are five main techniques to construct lateral wall aneurysms:

1. Non-ligated venous pouch with end-to-side anastomosis to the artery.
2. Non-ligated venous pouch with side-to-side anastomosis to the artery (variation of the former).
3. End-to-side anastomosis of the vein onto the artery with ligated venous pouch.
4. Side-to-side anastomosis of the vein onto the artery with ligated venous pouch.
5. End-to-side anastomosis of the venous pouch. The main advantage of this technique is the short-lasting clamping of the common carotid artery that thus avoids endothelial damage and vasospasm[21].

The main model for the construction of bifurcation aneurysms was performed using Forrest and O'Rielly's technique, in which the left common carotid artery of rabbits was partially anastomosed with the right common carotid artery. Next, a venous pouch (taken from the external jugular, anterior facial, or posterior facial vein) was grafted onto the knot formed by the union of the arterial anastomoses. The advantage of this technique was that unlike the lateral wall aneurysms, it did not induce aneurysmal thrombosis (**figure 3**)[24].

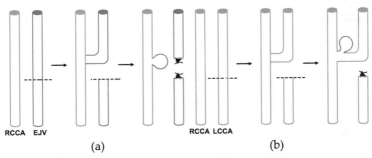

RCCA EJV   RCCA LCCA
(a)   (b)

Figure 3. Graphic representation of the main surgical models of experimental saccular aneurysm. (a) Lateral wall, (b) bifurcation (RCCA – right common carotid artery, EJV – external jugular vein, LCCA – left common carotid artery).

3.3.2. Other experimental models of aneurysms

In addition to the abovementioned techniques, other methods have been attempted to construct saccular aneurysms, such as hyper-flow (through the creation of arteriovenous fistulas), trauma (traumatic puncture of the arterial wall or using CO_2 laser), and chemical wall injury (by injecting nitrogen mustard or other substances directly inside the arterial wall) [51]. All of these techniques are less efficient than chemical induction and surgical construction. Despite these attempts at the construction of an experimental model of saccular aneurysm, none of these methods was able to reproduce all of the histopathological, geometric, and hemodynamic features of human intracranial saccular aneurysms [51-54]. Nevertheless, the enzymatic method has stood out in recent years.

3.3.3. Enzymatic models

3.3.3.1. Elastase-induced model

3.3.3.1.1. Mechanisms of action of elastase in aneurysm formation

The formation of saccular aneurysms depends on several mechanisms, including inflammatory reaction, weakening of the arterial wall, and hemodynamic tension. Enzymatic imbalance and inflammatory activity are some of the potential causes involved in aneurysm formation in humans. Anidjar (1992) perfused the abdominal aorta of a group of Wistar rats with pancreatic elastase from swine and used thioglycollate plus plasmin (activators of the inflammatory response) in another group of animals. Both groups exhibited an inflammatory reaction, elastic lamina fragmentation, and formation of fusiform aneurysms similar to those that occur in humans. The inflammatory activity was stronger in the elastase group (achieving its peak on the sixth day) and produced macrophages, polymorphonuclear cells, helper and suppressor T lymphocytes in the arterial wall. Combined with the progression of the inflammatory activity, the diameter of the abdominal aorta increased[55]. Halpern (1994) established the sequence and synchrony of induction of the inflammatory response. Elastase induces injury of the arterial wall, which triggers an initial inflammatory response. The inflammatory cells then activate endogenous proteinases (molecular weight between 50 and 90 kD) and the destruction of elastin and collagen, in addition to aortic dilation. Halpern's study showed that the rupture of elastin and its contact with macrophages are the main events in the activation of endogenous proteinases, which results in increased tissue destruction [56].

Although inflammatory activity might lead to destruction of the elastic fibers and a weakening of the arterial wall, its role in the development of saccular aneurysms has not been fully established. Other mechanisms may also participate in aneurysm formation such as alterations of the mechanical properties of arteries together with the hemodynamic tension on the vascular wall, which can produce aneurysms by themselves. Miskolczi (1997) demonstrated this phenomenon in an in vitro study, in which the common carotid arteries of swine and sheep were isolated and their walls were digested using pancreatic elastase from swine. Next, the arterial segments were placed between a pulsatile flow artificial pump and a series of test tubes, which allowed the control of variables such as flow, pulsation, and pressure without inducing the inflammatory response that occurs in in vivo studies. Consequently, small saccular aneurysms appeared at the sites where the elastin was damaged and hemodynamic tension was exerted on the weakened arterial wall[57].

3.3.3.1.2. Creation and improvement of the elastase-induced model

Based on studies of experimental aneurysm creation using elastase [55, 56], Cawley et al. (1996) developed a new experimental model of lateral wall aneurysms in rabbits. This model consisted of dissecting the neck of rabbits, ligating the proximal segment of the external carotid artery, and performing intra-arterial perfusion of pancreatic elastase from swine. Three weeks later, saccular aneurysms were formed, which, from angiographic and histological perspectives, were very similar to those in humans. However, the lumen remained patent in only 40% of the aneurysms, because lateral aneurysms do not originate from the type of hemodynamic stress and intra-aneurysmal blood flow that occur at the bifurcations of the human cerebral arteries[58].

Cloft et al. (1999) improved this model by producing greater hemodynamic stress on the left common carotid artery (LCCA), which was directly hit by the blood flow from the ascending aorta in two-thirds of the rabbits. This technique is fully endovascular and consists of insufflating a balloon at the origin of the LCCA and isolating a small arterial segment for intraluminal infusion of bovine pancreatic elastase for 30 minutes. Angiographic control was performed by the dissection and retrograde puncture of the femoral arteries. This method succeeded in producing aneurysms with an average size of 3.0 mm x 5.0 mm whose lumen remained patent up to three months after creation. From a microscopic point of view, all of the aneurysms exhibited intact endothelium, the absence of an inflammatory response, moderately damaged elastic lamina inside of the aneurysm (but undamaged at the neck), and apical thrombus. No animal exhibited neurological sequelae (due to the intracranial collateral vessels network) or showed systemic signs of elastase intoxication[59].

Kallmes et al. (1999) modified this method by creating additional hemodynamic tension on the proximal segment of the right common carotid artery (RCCA), which is located between the brachiocephalic artery and ascending aorta, and mimics a "bifurcation aneurysm." In addition, the long curvature of the brachiocephalic artery increased the hemodynamic tension at the origin of the RCCA compared to the LCCA. Further modification of this model consisted of reducing the time of enzymatic digestion to 20 minutes (**figure 4**).

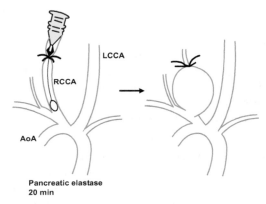

Figure 4. Graphic representation of the endovascular elastase-induced aneurysm construction technique. AoA – aortic arch, RCCA – right common carotid artery and LCCA – left common carotid artery. Modified from Hoh, 2004[60].

These technical modifications resulted in experimental aneurysms similar to those observed in humans with regard to the arterial origin, shape, hemodynamics, and patency. The high hemodynamic tension caused by the long curvature of the brachiocephalic artery makes these experimental aneurysms similar to those occurring in the ophthalmic segment of the human internal carotid artery[40]. Altes et al. (2000) used the RCCA for the intraluminal infusion of pancreatic elastase from swine in rabbits and obtained aneurysms in 89% of the animals. Two weeks later, the elastic lamina ruptured and aneurysms were formed (average dimensions of 4.5 mm x 7.5 mm), with organized thrombus in the aneurysm dome, whereas the elastic lamina was undamaged in the walls of the parent arteries. The cells present in the organized thrombus exhibited features of smooth muscle cells and fibroblasts. Ten weeks later, no significant alterations were observed. The execution of this technique required less than one hour, and although it included surgical procedures (e.g., section of the RCCA), this technique exhibited lower morbidity and mortality compared to the use of the LCCA[43].

From a technical perspective, it is noteworthy that the concentration of elastase and the time of incubation exert a partial effect on the size of the aneurysms. One study compared animals that were not subjected to elastase to animals that were subjected to low, medium, and high concentrations of this drug, under variable durations. The rabbits that were not subjected to elastase exhibited complete thrombosis of the arterial stump and did not form aneurysms, whereas the rabbits that were given elastase in progressive concentrations formed aneurysms. The increase of the elastase dose above a given value did not influence the size of the aneurysms; however, high concentrations of elastase induced the dilation of the parent artery and resulted in a more complex geometry of the aneurysm neck, which is closer to that observed in human aneurysms. Low concentration (25%) of elastase induced aneurysms without dilation of the adjacent artery[61].

Hoh et al. (2004) developed a simpler technique of construction and obtained aneurysms similar to those previously mentioned. The first simplification consisted of the use of a 24-gauge angiocatheter (instead of an introducer) and transitory occlusion of the origin of the RCCA using a neurosurgical clamp (instead of a balloon)[60]. The second simplification was achieved using an accurate neurological assessment of the rabbits using a four-point scale to rate the observed movements of the rabbits on a flat surface to verify whether paresis of the legs or abnormal gait occurred (movements in a circle or difficulty to walk). Accordingly, the animals were rated as grade I – no neurological deficit; grade II: minimal of suspected neurological deficit; grade III: mild neurological deficit without abnormal motion; and grade IV: remarkable neurological deficit and abnormal motion[62].

Although the studies performed to date have not reported any loss of animals, Möller-Hartmann et al. (2003) found a mortality of 25% due to the accidental passage of elastase into the superior thyroid artery with an aberrant origin or into the tracheoesophageal branch, which originated in the common carotid artery, resulting in hemorrhagic necrosis of the trachea[63]. Another source of undesirable distribution of elastase and tracheal necrosis is the anomalous origin of the tracheobronchial artery, which can be identified in angiographies as a small branch perpendicular to the proximal part of the RCCA, and runs medially towards the trachea[64]. Therefore, the elimination of those anomalous vessels (by ligation, coagulation or placing of the introducer lower inside the RCCA) is crucial for success in aneurysm creation by intraluminal infusion of elastase[63].

In addition to the problem posed by aberrant vessels, Krings et al. (2003) identified two additional potential causes of failure of the elastase model. The first potential cause depends on how elastase is injected through the introducer. Thus, instead of elastase, the blood column of the introducer dead space is pushed into the arterial lumen. Furthermore, the authors observed that doses of 100U of elastase were usually lethal. To address these problems, the authors reduced the dose of elastase to 20 U and performed a contrast injection test to detect aberrant arteries as follows: after occluding with a balloon in the proximal area of the RCCA, a non-ionic contrast material was injected (by means of an introducer) inside the RCCA, and the contrast column was verified for two minutes. If the contrast material remained, without washing out or dilution for two minutes, the test was deemed to be negative, i.e., there were no anomalous vessels. Otherwise, the test was deemed to be positive, and the introducer was advanced to a more proximal site of the RCCA where the contrast washing out or dilution no longer occurred. When these procedures were applied, none of the animals died, and all developed aneurysms. The full duration of this procedure was 40 minutes. The problem posed by the blood column and contrast material inside of the introducer was resolved by performing continuous suction using a syringe[65].

Prospective studies on the morphology and viability of elastase-induced aneurysms in rabbits require serial high-quality angiographic control. Three routes are currently used: the femoral arteries, left external auricular vein, and left central auricular artery. Miskolczi et al. (2005) suggested performing a retrograde puncture of the left central auricular artery as the best route, because the femoral artery is narrow and fragile and thus exhibits a high risk of injury and definitive loss. In addition, retrograde femoral catheterization requires the dissection of the groin, arteriotomy, and subsequent ligation with permanent vascular occlusion, thus making subsequent angiography at this site impossible. Puncture of the left external auricular vein allows for repeated injections of contrast material, but the resulting images exhibit low spatial resolution and frequent motion-related artifacts. In contrast, the left central auricular artery allows for repeated injections, high-quality images, and excellent visualization of the brachiocephalic trunk vessels because rabbits usually exhibit LCCA of bovine origin; thus, when the contrast material is injected into the left central auricular artery, the brachiocephalic trunk and its branches immediately become filled. When the LCCA originates directly from the aortic arch or from a common origin with the brachiocephalic trunk, but the angle is unfavorable, the contrast material only fills the distal aortic arch. The anatomy of approximately 70% - 80% of white New Zealand rabbits is favorable for retrograde injection in the left central auricular artery; therefore, pre-selection is important to exclude animals with unfavorable anatomy from studies[66].

3.3.3.1.3. Morphological and geometric features

The elastase model efficiently reproduces aneurysms similar to ones that occur in the ophthalmic segment of the human internal carotid artery with regard to width, height, neck size, and diameter of the parent artery. These characteristics were very well established by Short et al. (2001), who prospectively studied 40 rabbits and observed that the size of the aneurysmal cavities afforded by the elastase model was appropriate for preclinical tests of endovascular occlusion techniques and devices. The authors measured the width (points in the cavity exhibiting the maximal width), height (measurement of the aneurysmal dome to the mid-portion of a line connecting the proximal and distal portions of the aneurysm neck), neck (maximal diameter between the proximal and distal portions of the aneurysm orifice), the diameter of the parent artery (diameter of the artery just proximal to the aneurysm neck), and the dome/neck ratio (maximal dome width/neck width). In addition, they classified the aneurysms as small (2.0 mm – 4.9 mm), medium-sized (5.0 mm – 9.9 mm), or large (10.0 – 16.0 mm). Moreover, the neck was classified as small (< 4 mm) or wide (> 4 mm). Two weeks later, all of the animals had survived, none showed clinical evidences of neurological insult, and exhibited aneurysms at the apex of the long curve of the brachiocephalic artery, with an elongated shape, and a height greater than the width. Medium-sized (50%) and large (42.5%) aneurysms with small necks (55%) prevailed. The average width of the cavity was 4.1 ± 1.2 mm, which varied between 2.5 and 7.1 mm, and the average height was 8.8 ± 2.6 mm, which varied between 3.0 and 15.6 mm. A dome/neck ratio > 1 was observed in 50% of the aneurysms with an average value of 1.13 ± 0.5, and the average diameter of the parent artery was 4.3 ± 1.4 mm. Although these measures were similar to those of human aneurysms, they did not reproduce all of the corresponding morphological characteristics, which are difficult to quantify for many reasons[44].

Short-term follow-up of elastase-induced aneurysms showed that their dimensions increased gradually up to the end of the first month after creation and then become stable. The average measurements of the dome width and length at days 3 and 28 after induction were (3.2 ± 0.6 mm; 5.0 ± 0.9 mm) and (6.0 ± 1.3 mm; 10.0 ± 2.2 mm), respectively. Conversely, the aneurysms that were not incubated with elastase progressively retracted and formed thrombi inside. Because a millimeter-scale was used and the differences found were small, the authors considered the low resolution of intravascular angiography, radiographic projections used, and variations of the cardiac cycle that promoted different intra-aneurysmal pressures to be potential sources of variation and the lack of histological correlation to be a limitation of the study[67]. Ding et al. (2006) studied the long-term permeability of elastase-induced aneurysms and observed that the aneurysmal cavity remained patent and without thrombi for up to two years after creation and that after the first month, their dimensions (width, height, and neck width) did not exhibit significant variation [68].

The size of the neck has paramount importance when testing endovascular devices, as well as in the study of the physiopathology of aneurysms, and might be modified during the construction of experimental aneurysms. This finding was revealed by Ding et al. (2005), who observed that the size of the neck might be controlled by adjusting the position of the balloon during incubation with elastase. When the balloon is placed high, that is, half inside the proximal RCCA and half inside the subclavian and brachiocephalic arteries, the neck of the resulting aneurysms is narrow (< 4 mm). When the balloon is placed low, that is, exclusively inside of the subclavian and brachiocephalic arteries, the neck of the resulting aneurysms is wide (> 4 mm). The authors further observed that the position of the balloon did not influence the length of the aneurysms and that the balloons that were placed low did not always result in wide necks[69].

In addition to the low position of the balloon, the geometric relationship between the longest axis of the aneurysms and the axis of the parent artery played an important role in the determination of local hemodynamics and the final architecture of aneurysms. Onizuka et al. (2006) compared the angle formed by the longest axis of aneurysms and the axis of the parent artery immediately and three months after aneurysm construction. The authors found a positive correlation between the neck size and the dome height. In addition, the dome height was proportional to the angle formed by the brachiocephalic artery and the aneurysm neck. Therefore, the authors concluded that the larger the angle, the greater the hemodynamic stress caused by the blood flow on the distal neck and the aneurysm bottom[70].

The volume of elastase-induced aneurysms might also be adjusted by the position of the RCCA ligation so that high ligations might create relatively larger aneurysms compared to the ones produced by low ligations. Ding et al. (2007) prospectively studied the influence of the height of the RCCA ligation on the volume of aneurysms. Ligations were rated lower when the height of the ligation point was 10-mm away from the origin of the RCCA and high when the ligation point was 15-mm away from the origin of the RCCA. The same authors applied the formula for the volume of cylinders to calculate the volume of aneurysms because the shape of the created aneurysms was cylindrical. The aneurysms with higher ligations exhibited larger volumes (102.4 ± 54.8 mm³) compared to the ones with lower ligations (36.6 ± 26.8 mm³). In addition, the aneurysms with higher ligations exhibited larger dimensions such as the neck (3.3 ± 0.8 mm), width (3.7 ± 0.7 mm), and height (9.0 ± 1.7 mm). The authors attributed these results to a larger cavity space of aneurysms with higher ligation, in addition to probable greater hemodynamic stress on the aneurysms. Finally, according to those authors, no animals died due to the accidental passage of elastase (through aberrant vessels) in the case of aneurysms with higher ligation[69].

3.3.3.1.4. Histology

Abruzzo et al. (1998) compared the histological characteristics between lateral wall aneurysms (produced by means of elastase incubation in the external carotid artery of rabbits) and lateral wall aneurysms constructed by grafting a venous pouch onto the common carotid artery of pigs. Both experimental aneurysms were compared to human aneurysms with 5 – 10 mm of diameter (recently ruptured and obtained at autopsy), whose main characteristics included: 1) a complete absence of the internal elastic lamina in the aneurysms, and abrupt termination of the internal elastic lamina of the parent artery at the margins of the saccular orifice; 2) complete absence of the tunica media in the aneurysms and abrupt termination of the tunica media of the parent artery at the margins of the aneurysmal orifice; 3) absence of intramural inflammatory reaction in the aneurysms; 4) absence of neointimal fibromuscular proliferation; 5) a sac wall thickness of 51 μm and a neck thickness of 52 μm. In three out of the five studied aneurysms, one-third of the aneurysmal cavity was filled by a thrombus at different stages of organization and firmly adhered to the point of rupture. The elastase-induced aneurysms exhibited an abrupt termination of the internal elastic lamina at the margins of the saccular orifice, but the tunica medica was undamaged and continued into the interior of the saccular part of the aneurysms. The sac walls exhibited a mild to moderately inflammatory cellular (monocytes and neutrophils) response and a mild fibromuscular response. The thickness of the neck was 49 μm, and the thickness at the sac wall was 44 μm. An unorganized thrombus filled one-third of the aneurysmal cavity in two out of the four investigated rabbits. The aneurysms constructed using a venous pouch exhibited a well-developed elastic lamina, and the tunica media extended into the sac wall. The wall of the venous pouch contained remarkable inflammatory infiltrate (monocytes and neutrophils) and extreme degrees of fibromuscular proliferation completely across the aneurysm wall, resulting in a remarkable neointimal thickening and luminal narrowing. The thickness of the dome wall was 228 μm, and the thickness at the neck was 350 μm. Thus, the authors concluded that from a histological perspective, the elastase-induced aneurysms were the ones most similar to human aneurysms, in addition to exhibiting little spontaneous fibromuscular response compared to the surgical model with venous pouch grafting[71]. Accordingly, the elastase-induced model is currently used in tests for endovascular devices[39-42].

3.3.3.2. Papain-induced model

Although the damage of elastic fibers induced by swine pancreatic elastase resulted in experimental aneurysms similar to those appearing in the ophthalmic segment of the human internal carotid artery, they are small (<5 mm), which is not completely consistent with the actual clinical characteristics of human aneurysms, where the aneurysms are larger than 5 mm. To overcome this limitation, Chinese researchers tested an association between elastase and collagenase in the *in vitro* pre-digestion of an arterial pouch grafted onto the aortic arch of rabbits; however, that model exhibited a higher tendency to spontaneously rupture[72]. To produce saccular aneurysms larger than 5 mm, De Oliveira et al. (2011) infused the papain enzyme successfully inside the right common carotid artery of rabbits[73].

3.3.3.3. Mechanisms of action of papain

Papain is a cysteine-proteinase type of endolytic enzyme extracted from the latex of green papaya (*Carica papaya*). It weighs 23,000 Da , and its molecules form a single peptide chain with 211 amino acid residues that fold into two distinct parts, which are divided by a cleft that represents its active site[74]. In addition to papain, the latex contains three additional enzymes (chymopapain, caricain, and glycil endopeptidase), which together with papain represent 80% of the enzymatic fraction, where papain corresponds to the smallest enzymatic fraction (5-8%). Although purification of papain is usually performed using precipitation techniques, it remains contaminated by other proteases[75]. With regard to its enzymatic activity, papain is activated by the addition of substances such as cyanide, reduced glutathione, and sulfate and is inactivated by oxidants. The maximal enzymatic activity occurs with a pH between 5 and 7.5. With regard to its specificity, in addition to hydrolyzing several substances, papain exhibits strong esterase activity, which makes its scope of action even wider to the point of acting on the very same substrates as pancreatic proteolytic enzymes with esterase activity[76].

Regarding its biological effects, papain exhibits remarkable elastolytic properties and has been successfully used in the production of experimental lung emphysema in animals[77, 78]. In addition to digesting elastic fibers, papain is also able to destroy collagen. Junqueira (1980) studied the ability of papain to destroy the collagen fibers of several tissues (cartilage, bone, skin, and blood vessel) from several animal species, such as *Gallus gallus* (chicken), *Canis familiaris* (dog), *Oryctolagus cuniculus* (rabbit) and *Sus scrofa* (pig), and observed that the degree of collagen destruction varies according to the type of tissue[79]. Ionescu (1977) used papain to de-antigenize a venous heterograft to subsequently graft it onto the common carotid artery of dogs and observed that papain caused an excessive weakening of the graft with a tendency to form venous aneurysms. To overcome this problem, the author subjected the grafts to a previous treatment with formol to maintain their rigidity and flexibility and not form aneurysms[80].

With regard to commercial presentation, papain is found as raw latex (~ 12 U/mg), lyophilized powder (10 U/mg) and aqueous suspension (16-40 U/mg)[81].

3.3.3.4. Creation of papain-induced aneurysms

The technique applied in the construction of papain-induced aneurysms uses the right common carotid artery of rabbits and is fully surgical, based on the study by Hoh et al. However, this technique does not use angiography during the puncture of the right common carotid artery and injection of the enzyme. This simplification proved to be safe and efficacious, and no animal exhibited complications due to the unduly passage of papain to an aberrant vascular branch that was accidentally present in the neck of the animals. Other innovations were the removal of the aortic arch and the supra-aortic trunks, direct measurement of the macroscopic dimensions of aneurysms and vessels using a caliper, and quantitative histological studies by means of histomorphometry in addition to a qualitative histological analysis[60,73].

3.3.3.5. Morphologic and geometric features

Papain-induced aneurysms exhibited a size similar to the elastase-induced aneurysms described in previous studies. Nevertheless, it is noteworthy to stress that the papain-induced aneurysms were measured directly on the right common carotid artery. This is an important point because most of the studies performed using elastase employed digital subtraction angiography to measure the aneurysms, which led to an overestimate of the aneurysm size. Thus, if papain-induced aneurysms were also measured by means of digital subtraction angiography, then their size would have most likely been overestimated. Independent from the method used, papain was efficacious in producing saccular aneurysms with an average diameter of 3.8 +/- 1.4 mm (2.5-7.0 mm), similar to those appearing in the ophthalmic segment of the human internal carotid artery.

3.3.3.6. Histology

From a histological perspective, papain caused the destruction of elastic fibers, endothelial damage, thrombosis, and intimal fibrosis. These alterations are similar to those found in elastase-induced aneurysms, in which the only difference is the degree of thrombosis, which was more remarkable in the papain-induced aneurysms[73].

3.3.3.7. Future of the enzymatic model

Currently, there are no ideal animal models of experimental saccular aneurysms available. From a practical perspective, it is impossible for one single model to reproduce the full histological, geometric, and hemodynamic characteristics of the wide variety of aneurysms and human-related conditions. Nevertheless, the enzymatic model has been increasingly used in the production of saccular aneurysms due to its simplicity, easy execution, and lower cost, resulting from the use of small animals such as rabbits, in addition to allowing the control of height, width, and size of the aneurysm neck. Furthermore, the enzymatic model can be improved, as a wide variety of enzymes have not yet been tested. Despite the advantages of the enzymatic model, the use of both elastase and papain exhibits some limitations, such as an intramural inflammatory response, endothelial damage, and thrombosis. Indeed, thrombosis is the most important effect because it hinders the interpretation of the results of the embolization materials tested. However, even when they are present, the intra-aneurysmal thrombi do not invalidate this experimental model because under actual clinical conditions, most human aneurysms have thrombi present. Therefore, although they are not ideal for preclinical tests of embolization materials, enzymatic models most closely mimic the actual clinical conditions and thus exhibit a high potential to contribute to the study of the physiopathology of human intracranial aneurysms and testing of embolization materials and endovascular devices.

Author details

Ivanilson Alves de Oliveira
Neuroradiology, Experimental Medicine Laboratory, Universidade Federal de Sergipe-UFS, Brazil

4. References

[1]   Nyström H.S.M. Development of intracranial aneurysms as revealed by electron microscopy. J Neurosurg, 1963. 20: p. 329-337.

[2]   Rhoton A.L., Jr. Anatomy of saccular aneurysms. Surg Neurol, 1980. 14(1): p. 59-66.

[3]   Senegor M. Traumatic pericallosal aneurysm in a patient with no major trauma. Case report. J Neurosurg, 1991. 75(3): p. 475-7.

[4]   Barker C.S. Peripheral cerebral aneurysm associated with a glioma. Neuroradiology, 1992. 34(1): p. 30-2.

[5]   Frazee J.G., Cahan L.D. and Winter J. Bacterial intracranial aneurysms. J Neurosurg, 1980. 53(5): p. 633-41.

[6]   Lee K.S., Liu S.S., Spetzler R.F., Rekate H.L. Intracranial mycotic aneurysm in an infant: report of a case. Neurosurgery, 1990. 26(1): p. 129-33.

[7]   Bohmfalk G.L., Story J.L., Wissinger J.P., Brown, W.E. Bacterial intracranial aneurysm. J Neurosurg, 1978. 48(3): p. 369-82.

[8]   Brown R.D., Jr., Wiebers D.O. and Forbes G.S. Unruptured intracranial aneurysms and arteriovenous malformations: frequency of intracranial hemorrhage and relationship of lesions. J Neurosurg, 1990. 73(6): p. 859-63.

[9]   Brown B.M. and Soldevilla F. MR angiography and surgery for unruptured familial intracranial aneurysms in persons with a family history of cerebral aneurysms. AJR Am J Roentgenol, 1999. 173(1): p. 133-8.

[10] Schievink W.I., Parisi J.E, Piepgras D.G., Michels V.V. Intracranial aneurysms in Marfan's syndrome: an autopsy study. Neurosurgery, 1997. 41(4): p. 866-70; discussion 871.

[11] Heiserman J.E., Drayer B.P., Fram E.K., Keller P.J. MR angiography of cervical fibromuscular dysplasia. AJNR Am J Neuroradiol, 1992. 13(5): p. 1454-7.

[12] Kopitnik T.A. and Samson D.S. Management of subarachnoid haemorrhage. J Neurol Neurosurg Psychiatry, 1993. 56(9): p. 947-59.

[13] Dix G.A., Gordon W., Kaufmann A.M., Sutherland I.A., Sutherland G.R. Ruptured and unruptured intracranial aneurysms--surgical outcome. Can J Neurol Sci, 1995. 22(3): p. 187-91.

[14] Winn H.R., Almaani W.S., Berga S.L., Jane J.A., Richardson A.E. The long-term outcome in patients with multiple aneurysms. Incidence of late hemorrhage and implications for treatment of incidental aneurysms. J Neurosurg, 1983. 59(4): p. 642-51.

[15] Yasargil M.G. and Fox J.L. The microsurgical approach to intracranial aneurysms. Surg Neurol, 1975. 3(1): p. 7-14.

[16] Guglielmi G., Vinuela F., Dion J., Duckwiler G. Electrothrombosis of saccular aneurysms via endovascular approach. Part 2: Preliminary clinical experience. J Neurosurg, 1991. 75(1): p. 8-14.

[17] Derdeyn C.P., Barr J.D., Berenstein A., Connors J.J., Dion J.E., Duckwiler G.R., Higashida R.T., Strother C.M., Tomsick T.A., Turski P. The International Subarachnoid Aneurysm Trial (ISAT): a position statement from the Executive Committee of the American Society of Interventional and Therapeutic Neuroradiology and the American Society of Neuroradiology. AJNR Am J Neuroradiol, 2003. 24(7): p. 1404-8.

[18] Fagundes D.J., Taha M.O. Modelo animal de doença:critérios de escolha e espécies de animais de uso corrente. Acta Cirúrgica Brasileira, 2004. 19(1): p. 59-65.

[19] Hashimoto N., Handa H. and Hazama F. Experimentally induced cerebral aneurysms in rats. Surg Neurol, 1978. 10(1): p. 3-8.

[20] German W.J. and Black S.P.W. Experimental production of carotid aneurysms. N Engl J Med, 1954. 250(3): p. 104-6.

[21] Massoud T.F., Guglielmi G., Ji C., Vinuela F., Duckwiler G.R. Experimental saccular aneurysms. I. Review of surgically-constructed models and their laboratory applications. Neuroradiology, 1994. 36(7): p. 537-46.

[22] Schanaider A., Silva P.C., The use of animals in experimental surgery. Acta Cirúrgica Brasileira, 2004. 19(4): p. 1-9.

[23] Hashimoto N., Kim C., Kikuchi H., Kojima M., Kang Y., Hazama F. Experimental induction of cerebral aneurysms in monkeys. J Neurosurg, 1987. 67(6): p. 903-5.

[24] Forrest M.D. and O'Reilly G.V. Production of experimental aneurysms at a surgically created arterial bifurcation. AJNR Am J Neuroradiol, 1989. 10(2): p. 400-2.

[25] Hashimoto N., Handa H. and Hazama F. Experimentally induced cerebral aneurysms in rats: part II. Surg Neurol, 1979. 11(3): p. 243-6.

[26] Hashimoto N., Handa H. and Hazama F. Experimentally induced cerebral aneurysms in rats: Part III. Pathology. Surg Neurol, 1979. 11(4): p. 299-304.

[27] Kerber C.W. and Buschman R.W. Experimental carotid aneurysms: I. Simple surgical production and radiographic evaluation. Invest Radiol, 1977. 12(2): p. 154-7.

[28] Nagata I., Handa H. and Hashimoto N. Experimentally induced cerebral aneurysms in rats: part IV--cerebral angiography. Surg Neurol, 1979. 12(5): p. 419-24.

[29] Hashimoto N., Handa H. Nagata I., Hazama, F. Experimentally induced cerebral aneurysms in rats: Part V. Relation of hemodynamics in the circle of Willis to formation of aneurysms. Surg Neurol, 1980. 13(1): p. 41-5.

[30] Nagata I., Handa H., Hashimoto N., Hazama F. Experimentally induced cerebral aneurysms in rats: Part VI. Hypertension. Surg Neurol, 1980. 14(6): p. 477-9.

[31] Nakatani H., Hashimoto N., Kikuchi H., Yamaguchi S., Niimi H. In vivo flow visualization of induced saccular cerebral aneurysms in rats. Acta Neurochir (Wien), 1993. 122(3-4): p. 244-9.

[32] Stehbens W.E. Experimental production of aneurysms by microvascular surgery in rabbits. Vasc Surg, 1973. 7(3): p. 165-75.

[33] de los Reyes R.A., Boehm F.H., Boehm F.H., Ehler W., Kennedy D., Shagets F., Woodruff W., Smith T. Direct angioplasty of the basilar artery in baboons. Surg Neurol, 1990. 33(3): p. 185-91.

[34] Yoshino Y., Niimi Y., Song J.K., Khoyama S., Shin Y.S., Berenstein A. Endovascular treatment of intracranial aneurysms: comparative evaluation in a terminal bifurcation aneurysm model in dogs. J Neurosurg, 2004. 101(6): p. 996-1003.

[35] Graves V.B., Strother C.M., Partington C.R., Rappe A. Flow dynamics of lateral carotid artery aneurysms and their effects on coils and balloons: an experimental study in dogs. AJNR Am J Neuroradiol, 1992. 13(1): p. 189-96.

[36] Spetzger U., Reul J., Weis J., Bertalanffy H., Thron A., Gilsbach J.M. Microsurgically produced bifurcation aneurysms in a rabbit model for endovascular coil embolization. J Neurosurg, 1996. 85(3): p. 488-95.

[37] Spetzger U., Reul J., Weis J., Bertalanffy H., Gilsbach J.M. Endovascular coil embolization of microsurgically produced experimental bifurcation aneurysms in rabbits. Surg Neurol, 1998. 49(5): p. 491-4.

[38] Raymond J., Salazkin I., Metcalfe A., Robledo O., Gevry G., Roy D., Weill A., Guilbert F. Lingual artery bifurcation aneurysms for training and evaluation of neurovascular devices. AJNR Am J Neuroradiol, 2004. 25(8): p. 1387-90.

[39] Kallmes D.F., Helms G.A., Hudson S.B., Altes T.A., Do H.M., Mandell J.W., Cloft H.J. Histologic evaluation of platinum coil embolization in an aneurysm model in rabbits. Radiology, 1999. 213(1): p. 217-22.

[40] Kallmes D.F., Williams A.D., Cloft H.J., Lopes M.B., Hankins G.R., Helm G.A. Platinum coil-mediated implantation of growth factor-secreting endovascular tissue grafts: an in vivo study. Radiology, 1998. 207(2): p. 519-23.

[41] Hans F.J., Krings T., Möller-Hartmann W., Thiex R., Pfeffer J., Cherer K., Brunn A., Dreeskamp H., Stein K.P., Meetz A., Gilsbach J.M., Thron A. Endovascular treatment of experimentally induced aneurysms in rabbits using stents: a feasibility study. Neuroradiology, 2003. 45(7): p. 430-4.

[42] Struffert T., Roth C., Romeike B., Grunwald I.O., Reith W. Onyx in an experimental aneurysm model: histological and angiographic results. J Neurosurg, 2008. 109(1): p. 77-82.

[43] Altes T.A., Cloft H.J., Short J.G., DeGast A., Do H.M., Helm G.A., Kallmes D.F. 1999 ARRS Executive Council Award. Creation of saccular aneurysms in the rabbit: a model suitable for testing endovascular devices. American Roentgen Ray Society. AJR Am J Roentgenol, 2000. 174(2): p. 349-54.

[44] Short J.G., Fujiwara N.H., Marx W.F., Helm G.A., Cloft H.J., Kallmes D.F. Elastase-induced saccular aneurysms in rabbits: comparison of geometric features with those of human aneurysms. JNR Am J Neuroradiol, 2001. 22(10): p. 1833-7.

[45] Adams D.F., Olin T.B. and Redman H.C. Catheterization of Arteries in the Rabbit. Radiology, 1965. 84: p. 531-5.

[46] Angel-James J. Variations in the vasculature of the aortic arch and its major branches in the rabbit. Acta Anat, 1974. 87: p. 283-300.

[47] Bugge J. Arterial supply of the cervical viscera in the rabbit. Acta Anat (Basel), 1967. 68(2): p. 216-27.

[48] Blanding J.D., Jr., Ogilvie R.W., Hoffman C.L., Knisely W.H. The Gross Morphology of the Arterial Supply to the Trachea, Primary Bronchi, and Esophagus of the Rabbit. Anat Rec, 1964. 148: p. 611-4.

[49] Du Boulay G.H. Comparative neuroradiologic vascular anatomy of experimental animals. In: Newton D.G. and Potts T.H. (ed.) Radiology of the skull and brain. Saint Louis: Mosby; 1974. p. 2763-86.

[50] Chungcharoen D., Daly M.B.; Neil E. The efect of occlusion upon the intrasinusal presure with special reference to vascular communications between the carotid and vertebral circulations in the dog, cat, and rabbit. J Physiol, 1952. 117: p. 56-76.

[51] Stehbens W.E. Evaluation of aneurysm models, particularly of the aorta and cerebral arteries. Exp Mol Pathol, 1999. 67(1): p. 1-14.

[52] Nishikawa M., Smith R.D. and Yonekawa Y. Experimental intracranial aneurysms. Surg Neurol, 1977. 7(4): p. 241-4.

[53] TerBrugge K.G., Lasjaunias P. and Hallacq P. Experimental models in interventional neuroradiology. AJNR Am J Neuroradiol, 1991. 12(6): p. 1029-33.

[54] Powell J. Models of arterial aneurysm: for the investigation of pathogenesis and pharmacotherapy--a review. Atherosclerosis, 1991. 87(2-3): p. 93-102.

[55] Anidjar S., Dobrin P.B., Eichorst M., Graham G.P., Chejfec G. Correlation of inflammatory infiltrate with the enlargement of experimental aortic aneurysms. J Vasc Surg, 1992. 16(2): p. 139-47.

[56] Halpern V.J., Nackman G.B., Gandhi R.H., Irizzary E., Scholes J.V., Ramey, W.G. The elastase infusion model of experimental aortic aneurysms: synchrony of induction of endogenous proteinases with matrix destruction and inflammatory cell response. J Vasc Surg, 1994. 20(1): p. 51-60.

[57] Miskolczi L., Guterman L.R., Flaherty J.D., Hpkins L.N. Saccular aneurysm induction by elastase digestion of the arterial wall: a new animal model. Neurosurgery, 1998. 43(3): p. 595-600; discussion 600-1.

[58] Cawley C.M., Dawson R.C., Shengelaia G., Bonner G., Barrow D.L., Colohan A.R. Arterial saccular aneurysm model in the rabbit. AJNR Am J Neuroradiol, 1996. 17(9): p. 1761-6.

[59] Cloft H.J., Altes T.A., MArx W.F., Raible R.J., Hudson S.B., Helm G.A., Mandell J.W. Jensen M.E., Dion J.E., Kallmes D.F., Endovascular creation of an in vivo bifurcation aneurysm model in rabbits. Radiology, 1999. 213(1): p. 223-8.

[60] Hoh B.L., Rabinov J.D., Pryor J.C., Ogilvy C.S. A modified technique for using elastase to create saccular aneurysms in animals that histologically and hemodynamically resemble aneurysms in human. Acta Neurochir (Wien), 2004. 146(7): p. 705-11.

[61] Kallmes D.F., Fujiwara N.H., Berr S.S., Helm G.A., Cloft H.J. Elastase-induced saccular aneurysms in rabbits: a dose-escalation study. AJNR Am J Neuroradiol, 2002. 23(2): p. 295-8.

[62] Endo S., Branson P.J. and Alksne J.F. Experimental model of symptomatic vasospasm in rabbits. Stroke, 1988. 19(11): p. 1420-5.

[63] Möller-Hartmann W., Krings T., Stein K.P., Dreeskamp A., Meetz A., Thiex R., Hans F.J., Gilsbach J.M., Thron A. Aberrant origin of the superior thyroid artery and the tracheoesophageal branch from the common carotid artery: a source of failure in elastase-induced aneurysms in rabbits. AJR Am J Roentgenol, 2003. 181(3): p. 739-41.

[64] Thiex R., Hans F.J., Krings T., Möller-Hartmann W., Brunn A., Scherer K., Gilsbach J.M., Thron A. Haemorrhagic tracheal necrosis as a lethal complication of an aneurysm model in rabbits via endoluminal incubation with elastase. Acta Neurochir (Wien), 2004. 146(3): p. 285-9; discussion 289.

[65] Krings T., Möller-Hartmann W., Hans F.J., Thiex R., Brunn A., Scherer K., Meetz A., Dreeskamp H., Stein K.P., Gilsbach J.M., Thron A. A refined method for creating saccular aneurysms in the rabbit. Neuroradiology, 2003. 45(7): p. 423-9.

[66] Miskolczi L., Nemes B., Cesar L., Masanari O. Gounis M. Contrast injection via the central artery of the left ear in rabbits: a new technique to simplify follow-up studies. AJNR Am J Neuroradiol, 2005. 26(8): p. 1964-6.

[67] Fujiwara N.H., Cloft H.J., Marx W.F., Short J.G., Jensen M.E., Kallmes D.F. Serial angiography in an elastase-induced aneurysm model in rabbits: evidence for progressive aneurysm enlargement after creation. AJNR Am J Neuroradiol, 2001. 22(4): p. 698-703.

[68] Ding Y.H., Dai D., Lewis D.A., Danielson M.A., Kadirvel R., Cloft H.J., Kallmes D.F. Long-term patency of elastase-induced aneurysm model in rabbits. AJNR Am J Neuroradiol, 2006. 27(1): p. 139-41.

[69] Ding Y.H., Dai D., Danielson M.A., Kadirvel R., Lewis D.A., Cloft H.J., Kallmes D.F. Control of aneurysm volume by adjusting the position of ligation during creation of elastase-induced aneurysms: a prospective study. AJNR Am J Neuroradiol, 2007. 28(5): p. 857-9.

[70] Onizuka M., Miskolczi L., Gounis M.J., Seong J., Lieber B.B., Wakhloo A.K. Elastase-induced aneurysms in rabbits: effect of postconstruction geometry on final size. AJNR Am J Neuroradiol, 2006. 27(5): p. 1129-31.

[71] Abruzzo T., Shengelaia G.G., Dawson R.C., Owens D.S., Cawley C.M., Gravanis M.B. Histologic and morphologic comparison of experimental aneurysms with human intracranial aneurysms. AJNR Am J Neuroradiol, 1998. 19(7): p. 1309-14.

[72] Yang X.J., Li L. and Wu Z.X. A novel arterial pouch model of saccular aneurysm by concomitant elastase and collagenase digestion. J Zhejiang Univ Sci B, 2007. 8(10): p. 697-703.

[73] de Oliveira I.A., Mendes Pereira Caldas J.G., Oliveira H.A., Brito E.A.C. Development of a new experimental model of saccular aneurysm by intra-arterial incubation of papain in rabbits. Neuroradiology, 2011. 53(11): p. 875-81.

[74] Drenth J., Jansonius J.N., Koekoek R., Swen H.M., Wolthers B.G. Structure of papain. Nature, 1968. 218(5145): p. 929-32.

[75] Nitsawang S., Hatti-Kaul R., Kanarawud P., Purification of papain from Carica papaya latex: aquous two-phase extraction versus two-step salt precipitation. Enzime and Microbiolol technology., 2006: p. 1-5.

[76] Kimmel J.R., Smith E.L. Crystaline papain. I. Preparation,specificity and activation. J Biol Chem, 1954. 207(2): p. 515-531.

[77] Johanson W.G., Jr. and Pierce A.K. Effects of elastase, collagenase, and papain on structure and function of rat lungs in vitro. J Clin Invest, 1972. 51(2): p. 288-93.

[78] Gross P., Babyak M.A., Tolker E., Kaschak M. Enzymatically Produced Pulmonary Emphysema; a Preliminary Report. J Occup Med, 1964. 6: p. 481-4.

[79] Junqueira L.C., Bignolas G., Mourão P.A.S., Bonetti S.S., Quantitation of collagen - proteoglycan interaction in tissue sections. Connect Tissue Res, 1980. 7(2): p. 91-6.

[80] Ionescu G., Neumann E., Domokos M., Andercou A., Cardan E., Cucu A. Experimental preparation of deantigenized vascular heterografts and study of tolerance after transplantation. Acta Chir Belg, 1977. 76(4): p. 393-9.

[81] Sigma-Aldrich. Reagentes bioquímicos e kits para pesquisa em ciências da vida. Sigma-Aldrich (ed.); Brasil. 2006:p. 1812-1813.

Chapter 3

Mineral Components in Aneurysms

Katarzyna Socha and Maria H. Borawska

Additional information is available at the end of the chapter

1. Introduction

Some studies reported imbalance of mineral components in patients with aneurysms [1-5]. The single available scientific reports from recent years describe the effect of certain dietary factors on the risk of aneurysm, such as eating high-cholesterol, fatty meat, alcohol consumption, inadequate intake of fruits and vegetables and also smoking. According to the authors of these papers it results in an increased incidence of aortic and cerebral aneurysms [6-9].

The objective of our research was investigation the relationships between content of selected mineral components: magnesium (Mg), copper (Cu), zinc (Zn), selenium (Se), lead (Pb) and cadmium (Cd) and dietary habits and smoking in patients with abdominal aortic aneurysm (AAA) and cerebral aneurysm (CA). We compared the status of examined elements in patients with aneurysm and healthy people in similar age (control group).

2. Material and methods

We examined 4 groups:

1. Patients with AAA (45 men and 5 women) aged 42-81 years, hospitalized at the Department of Vascular Surgery and Transplantology of Medical University of Bialystok, from which blood samples were taken. The samples of aortic wall and parietal thrombus were collected during surgery. The study included patients with an aneurysm diameter of 3.5 - 15 cm. In 33% of patients occurred aneurysm rupture, in 37% was inflammatory aneurysm, and in 45% of patients femoral artery aneurysm coexisted;

2. Patients with CA (27 men and 43 women) aged 16 - 73 years, hospitalized at the Department of Neurosurgery of Medical University of Bialystok, from which blood samples were taken in the early phase (up to 72 hrs.) after the aneurysmal rupture;

3. Healthy people (n = 22), appropriately matched to examined groups by age and gender, from which blood samples were taken – control group;
4. Aortic wall samples (n = 15) without aneurysm, taken from died people aged 39 – 79 years – control group.

Food-frequency questionnaires were implemented to collect the dietary data. The patients with aneurysms were asked to complete the questionnaire concerning the consumption frequency of food product and smoking by the National Food and Nutrition Institute and the National Cardiology Institute [10]. 28 patients with CA, due to poor health were disclosed from nutritional information collecting. The list of food commodities consisted of 36 food items (white bread, wholegrain bread, sweets, cereal products, grain products, pulses, milk, cottage cheese, other sorts of cheese, meat, poultry, offal, sausages, ham, meat products, bacon, tinned meat, tinned fish, fresh fish, eggs, butter, margarine, vegetable oils, potatoes, processed vegetables, fresh vegetables, fruit, sugar added to beverages, marmalade, honey, soft drinks, beer, wine, vodka, coffee, tea). The consumption frequency of different kind of food was estimated according to the following criteria: frequent consumption was defined as an intake of certain food products twelve to thirty days per month, except fish, that was eaten four to twelve a month. Food products eaten less frequently were classified into "sporadic consumption" group.

The concentration of mineral components in deproteinated blood and tissues, after microwave mineralization in concentrated nitric acid, was analyzed by flame (Mg, Zn) and electrothermal (Cu, Se, Pb, Cd) atomic absorption spectrometry method with Zeeman-effect background correction on Z-5000 and Z-2000 instrument (Hitachi). Certified reference materials: Seronorm – human serum and whole blood, BCR184 – bovine muscle were used to test the accuracy of this methods. The results of the quality control analyses were in agreement with reference values. The Department of Bromatology participates in a quality control program of the estimation of trace elements of the National Institute of Public Health and Institute of Nuclear Chemistry and Technology.

Statistical analyses were performed using Statistica v. 9.1 software. Differences between independent groups were tested by the Mann-Whitney U-test. The correlations were calculated and tested by the Spearman rank test. For estimation the influence of dietary habits on content of mineral components in the examined patients we have used multiple linear regression analysis. Values of $p < 0.05$ were considered to be significantly different.

3. Results and discussion

3.1. Magnesium (Mg)

Mg as an activator of adenylate cyclase and ATPase cofactor is involved in most of the processes of the body. It participates in the synthesis and break-up of high-energy compounds, mainly ATP, activates enzymes involved in the metabolism of carbohydrates and fats, and is involved in protein synthesis [11]. Studies showed the efficacy of the compounds of Mg in the prevention and treatment of cardiovascular and nervous system, diabetes and some cancers, such as in the case of prostate cancer [12]. Mg decreases blood lipids, dilates blood vessels, reduces sensitivity to endogenous catecholamines, prevents hypercoagulability and reduces the sensitivity of the myocardium to hypoxia and also has anti-arrhythmic activity. In animal studies it was found that the deficiency of Mg causes hypercholesterolemia, hypertriglyceridemia and atherosclerosis [13]. Mg is one of the factors that modify the biosynthesis and degradation of elastin and collagen [14].

The average concentration of Mg in serum of patients with AAA was 21.88 ± 2.52 mg/L and did not differ significantly from the contents of this element in serum of healthy people: 21.09 ± 1.97 mg/L. The average content of Mg in the aortic wall with aneurysm: 191.40 ± 106.37 µg/g was significantly lower (p <0.03) compared to the concentration of this element in normal aorta - average: 299.15 ± 234.98 µg/g (Table 1). The average content of Mg in the parietal thrombus was 47.63 ± 11.93 µg/g. There was no significant correlation between the content of Mg in examined tissues. We found that cigarette smoking decrease concentration of Mg in parietal thrombus of patients with AAA [15].

The average concentration of Mg in serum of patients with CA was 21.26 ± 3.10 mg/L and did not differ significantly (p = 0.368) on the content of this element in the serum of healthy people: 20.62 ± 2.06 mg/L - Table 1 [16].

Type of aneurysm	Concentration of Mg (average ± SD)		p
AAA	Serum (mg/L)		$p_{1/2} = 0.110$
	1. Control group (n = 22)	2. Examined group (n = 49)	
	21.09 ± 1.97	21.88 ± 2.52	
	Aortic wall (µg/g)		$p_{3/4} < 0.03$
	3. Without aneurysm (n = 14)	4. With aneurysm (n = 49)	
	299.15 ± 234.98	$191.40 \pm 106.37 \downarrow$	
CA	Serum (mg/L)		$p_{5/6} = 0.368$
	5. Control group (n = 22)	6. Examined group (n = 65)	
	20.62 ± 2.06	21.26 ± 3.10	

SD – standard deviation, p – significance level, n – number of samples

Table 1. Concentration of Mg in patients with abdominal aortic aneurysm (AAA), cerebral aneurysm (CA) and in the control groups.

One of the factors that eliminate the development of the aneurysm may be proper diet [6-9], including adequate supply of mineral components, which are essential factors in numerous metabolic processes functioning as coenzymes or biologically active substances. Mg is absorbed from diet in about 50%, and there are many factors causing the negative balance of this element in the body. The source of Mg in the diet are: buckwheat, soya flour, cocoa, chocolate, seeds of legumes, spinach, wholegrain bread, nuts, figs, bananas, leafy vegetables, rice and fish [17].

Multiple regression analysis revealed a significant effect the dietary habits on Mg concentration in patients with the aneurysm. Dietary habits in about 50% (R^2 = 0.50) affected the concentration of Mg in the serum of the patients. Frequent consumption of fish and canned fish, grits, rice and legumes had the greatest influence on Mg status, but eating white bread, sweets and sugar was inversely correlated with concentration of Mg. A similar correlation in the case of frequent consumption of sweet bakery products and sweets we found in previous studies assessing the concentration of Mg in patients with larynx cancer [18]. It is known that one reason for the negative balance of Mg in the system are diabetes and eating foods rich in sugar [17]. Analysis of the Spearman rank correlation showed that people often consumed white bread (which significantly decreased serum Mg levels) did not consume wholegrain bread (r = - .327, p <0.05), which is a good source of Mg.

3.2. Copper (Cu)

Imbalance in the concentrations of mineral elements in the human body is regarded as one of the risk factors for cardiovascular disease. The biological role of copper (Cu) is related to its participation in the structures and functions of many enzymes (tyrosinase, cytochrome c oxidase, Cu / Zn - superoxide dismutase, an antioxidant and anti-inflammatory). The role of Cu in the inflammation process has not been clearly defined. Significance for this process is its participation in the synthesis of prostaglandins in the arachidonic acid cascade. However, the greatest importance in influencing Cu in the inflammatory process has control of the synthesis of oxygen free radicals, resulting from the presence of this element in superoxide dismutase. In chronic inflammatory process associated with a severe phagocytosis generated free radical compounds that lead to tissue damage. Particularly susceptible to free radical attack are polyunsaturated fatty acids, which are then oxidized. This leads to damage of biological membranes and increase their permeability. Cu reducing the release of lysosomal enzymes by oxidation of membrane thiols to disulfides, to decrease the permeability of biological membranes. Cu also affects the inflammatory process by connecting to histamine, resulting in a decrease of its activity. This trace mineral plays an active role in the synthesis of collagen, elastin, myelin formation, affects bone formation and erythropoiesis [19]. The changes in the Cu content in the arterial wall are important because deficiency of this element may impair the formation of cross-links in collagen and elastin molecules, and thus cause a weakening of the elastic properties of elastin and collagen mechanical resistance and to increase the solubility of these proteins [20]. Cu promotion of angiogenesis is well documented. Cu stimulates endothelial cell proliferation and differentiation and promotes microtubule formation in cultured saphenous veins [21]. The enzyme lysyl oxidase (LOX) is a copper-dependent extracellular enzyme that catalyzes lysine-derived cross-links in collagen and elastin. LOX-mediated cross-linking of collagen types I and III fibrils leads to the formation of stiff collagen types I and III fibers and their subsequent tissue deposition. Evidence from experimental and clinical studies shows that the excess of LOX is associated with an increased collagen cross-linking and stiffness [22]. It has been suggested that ceruloplasmin, which binds more than 90% Cu contained in human plasma and delivers Cu ions play an important role in the oxidative modification of low density lipoprotein (LDL). LDL contributes to the arising and development of atherosclerotic lesions in the arterial wall [23]. It was found that Cu is essential for the initiation of endothelial cell proliferation by the activation of angiogenic factors. Carcinogenic properties of Cu may also be related to its ability to bind to some proteins, giving them angiogenic activity [24].

The average concentration of Cu in serum of patients with AAA: 1.16 ± 0.36 mg/L was significantly higher (p <0.03) compared to the control group: 0.96 ± 0.16 mg/L (Table 2). The average content of Cu in the aneurysmal wall was 0.92 ± 0.36 µg/g, while in the parietal thrombus 1.50 ± 0.92 µg/g. We observed a significant correlation (correlation coefficient: r = 0.453, p <0.012) between the content of Cu in the aortic wall and parietal thrombus in patients with AAA [25].

Our new research showed that average content of Cu in serum of patients with CA was significantly (p<0.00003) lower (0.777 ± 0.32 mg/L) than in the control group (1.132 ± 0.41 mg/L) - Table 2. Imbalance in the concentration of Cu in the case of aneurysms have also been observed by other authors [1-2,4,5].

Type of aneurysm	Concentration of Cu (average ± SD)			p
	Serum (mg/L)			
TAB	1. Control group (n = 18)		2. Examined group (n = 34)	$p_{1/2} < 0.03$
	0.96 ± 0.16		1.16 ± 0.36 ↑	
CA	3. Control group (n = 22)		4. Examined group (n = 78)	$p_{3/4} < 0.00003$
	1.132 ± 0.41		0.777 ± 0.32 ↓	

SD – standard deviation, p – significance level, n – number of samples

Table 2. Concentration of Cu in patients with abdominal aortic aneurysm (AAA), cerebral aneurysm (CA) and in the control groups.

Dietary sources for Cu include whole grain cereals, legumes and green leafy vegetables, nuts, potatoes, oysters and other seafood, offal, poultry, cocoa, dried fruits such as prunes, raisins and yeast [26].

The increase of Cu concentration correlated positively with frequent consumption of ham, wholegrain products and negatively with frequent consumption of offal, probably due to higher concentrations of toxic elements in these products and their interactions [27].

3.3. Zinc (Zn)

The importance of zinc (Zn) in the human body is associated with its multidirectional biological activity by taking part in over 300 enzymatic reactions and metabolic disorders. Zn is a stabilizer or a catalyst for more than 200 enzymes that are involved in the processes of cellular respiration, protein and carbohydrate metabolism [28]. The most important biological role of Zn is to participate in the metabolism of nucleic acids and protein synthesis as an essential component of RNA and DNA polymerases [29]. Zn is involved in the metabolism of fatty acids n-3 prostaglandins, which, depending on the type and concentration may act anti-inflammatory, dilate blood vessels, lower blood pressure, prevent clotting, inhibit the synthesis of triglycerides and are essential in regulating the activity of T cells [30]. Zn is a protective factor in the structure and functioning of cell membranes, is involved in gene expression and cell differentiation. Due to the stabilizing properties of a protective effect on the integrity of the endothelial cell layer, which protects against harmful substances such as inflammatory cytokines and an excess of polyunsaturated fatty acids. It is suggest that an anti-arteriosclerosis role of Zn is related to prevention of this particular factors [31,32]. Zn also participates in the synthesis of collagen [33]. Due to antioxidant activity and anti-inflammatory properties Zn possesses anticancer activity. It was found that Zn supplementation has a beneficial effect on the reduction of angiogenesis and induction of inflammatory cytokines while increasing apoptosis in tumor cells [34,35]. Zn decreases absorption of Cu by competing for binding to metallothionein [36].

The average concentration of Zn in the serum of patients with AAA (0.653 ± 0.271 mg/L) was significantly lower (p <0.00007) than the level of Zn in serum in the control group: 0.996 ± 0.260 mg/L. The average content of Zn in the aortic wall with aneurysm was 21.157 ± 12.582 µg/g, whereas in normal aorta: 23.318 ± 14.038 µg/g (Table 3). The average concentration of Zn in the parietal thrombus was 10.622 ± 6.799 µg/g There was no significant correlation between the content of Zn in examined tissues [37].

The average concentration of Zn in the serum of patients with CA was significantly (p <0.03) lower (0.651 ± 0.20 mg/L) compared to the concentration of Zn in the serum of healthy subjects (0.761 ± 0.19 mg/L) - Table 3. We also showed that the level of Zn in the serum of patients who died during hospitalization was significantly (p <0.05) lower (0.544 ± 0.19 mg/L) compared to the concentration of Zn in the serum of patients who survived (0.684 ± 0 20 mg/L). There was a significantly (p <0.003) higher concentrations of Zn in serum of males (0.875 ± 0.17 mg/L) compared to the level of serum Zn in females (0.648 ± 0.13 mg/L) [38].

The absorption of Zn from food ranges from 10-40%. The diet and age have influence on the bioavailability of Zn. Excess of calcium, copper, iron and selenium in the diet decreases the bioavailability. Phytic acid and dietary fiber, found in plant food decrease its absorption, but amino acids increase the bioavailability of Zn. Food of animal origin (pork, poultry, fish, shellfish, oysters, offal, eggs, cheese) is one of the best sources of easily absorbed Zn. Plant products such as sunflower and pumpkin seeds, nuts, cereals with wholegrain bread, legume seeds, brown rice, onion, garlic and some mushrooms are also good sources of Zn [32,39,40].

Zn content significantly increased the frequent consumption of fish, canned fish and wholegrain breads, and decreased the frequent consumption of raw vegetables - probably due to the presence of these compounds impair the bioavailability [37,38,40].

Type of aneurysm	Concentration of Zn (average ± SD)		p
AAA	Serum (mg/L)		$p_{1/2} < 0.00007$
	1. Control group (n = 16)	2. Examined group (n = 42)	
	0.996 ± 0.260	0.653 ± 0.271↓	
	Aortic wall (µg/g)		$p_{3/4} = 0.650$
	3. Without aneurysm (n = 9)	4. With aneurysm (n = 42)	
	23.318 ± 14.038	21.157 ± 12.582	
CA	Serum (mg/L)		$p_{5/6} < 0.003$
	5. Control group (n = 22)	6. Examined group (n = 57)	
	0.761 ± 0.19	0.651 ± 0.20 ↓	

SD – standard deviation, p – significance level, n – number of samples

Table 3. Concentration of Zn in patients with abdominal aortic aneurysm (AAA), cerebral aneurysm (CA) and in the control groups.

3.4. Selenium (Se)

Se is a micronutrient essential to maintain normal physiological functions, but also has an excess of adverse effects on the body. Se content in food, and consequently in the body, is dependent on its presence in the environment. Poland is one of the regions with low content of Se in soil and its overdose of food practically does not happen. More common is deficiency of this micronutrient [41,42]. So far, about 20 selenoprotein, including glutathione peroxidase, selenoproteins P and W, iodothyronine deiodinase type 1,2 and 3, thioredoxin reductase, synthetase have been described [43]. Se is contained in the active center of glutathione peroxidase (GSH-Px) protecting the body against free radicals because of immunological and anti-inflammatory activities. Deficiency of Se can lead to cardiomyopathy and myocardial infarction, muscular dystrophy and fibrosis of pancreas [44]. Se is the element entered by selenocysteine into the genetic code and its low concentration may influence the increased risk of cancer (breast cancer, lung cancer) [45-48]. The metabolism of Se in the brain is different than in other organs - deficiency of this element causes accumulation of increasing quantities of Se in brain. Although the function of many selenoproteins are not yet exactly known, an important role of Se in the functioning of the brain in its normal development and disease states, such as schizophrenia, Parkinson's or Alzheimer's disease is suggested [49]. Se also shows a detoxifying effect in the case of exposure to toxic elements such as lead and cadmium; these metal ions readily form stable connection in a complex of poorly soluble selenides excluding those elements from the biochemical processes and improving their elimination from the body [44].

The average Se level in serum of patients with AAA (60.37 ± 21.2 µg/L) was significantly ($p < 0.008$) lower than in healthy volunteers (75.87 ± 22.4 µg/L). The average serum Se concentration in the examined group was below the reference range, which is 70-140 µg/L [50]. We have not found differences between the content of Se in the aortic wall of patients with AAA (52.31 ± 47.1 ng/g) and the control group: 55.44 ± 34.4 ng/g (died people) - Table 4. The average concentration of Se in parietal thrombus was 139.82 ± 44.6 ng/g. We have observed a significant correlation ($r = 0.69$, $p < 0.0001$) between the content of Se in serum and the parietal thrombus of examined patients. We observed a significantly lower ($p < 0.05$) concentration of Se in aortic wall of smoking than non-smoking patients [51].

The concentrations of Se in the serum of patients with CA (73.248 ± 13.30 µg/L) were similar to the average content of Se in the control group (75.789 ± 22.07 µg/L) - Table 4 [52].

Type of aneurysm	Concentration of Se (average ± SD)			p
AAA	Serum (µg/L)			$p_{1/2} < 0.008$
	1. Control group (n = 22)		2. Examined group (n = 49)	
	75.87 ± 22.4		60.37 ± 21.2 ↓	
	Aortic wall (ng/g)			$p_{3/4} = 0.839$
	3. Without aneurysm (n = 17)		4. With aneurysm (n = 40)	
	55.44 ± 34.4		52.31 ± 47.1	
CA	Serum (µg/L)			$p_{5/6} = 0.579$
	5. Control group (n = 22)		6. Examined group (n = 38)	
	75.79 ± 22.1		73.25 ± 13.3	

SD – standard deviation, p – significance level, n – number of samples

Table 4. Concentration of Se in patients with abdominal aortic aneurysm (AAA), cerebral aneurysm (CA) and in the control groups.

The content of Se in the diet depends on its content in foods. High-protein products such as meat, meat offal, fish, eggs and poultry are good sources of Se. Additionally plant foods like nuts (especially Brazil), tomatoes, cucumbers, onions, garlic, broccoli, cabbage, wheat germ, wholegrain cereals are also good sources of Se [44].

The frequent consumption of raw vegetables significantly increased the concentration of Se, which is consistent with the literature because it is known that the plant food, in which Se is present as a selenomethionine and selenocysteine, characterized by a higher bioavailability compared to animal products [44,53]. In addition frequent consumption of wholegrain bread, grits, rice, meat products, ham, poultry, eggs and honey increased levels of Se in the patients. Eggs, especially egg yolk and poultry in our country are a significant source of Se due to the addition of Se compounds to feed. We estimated the content of Se in different meats and the highest content of Se was in the poultry [54]. The consumption of offal, canned meat, vodka and wine was inversely correlated with Se concentration in examined patients. It is known that alcohol impairs the absorption of minerals; sulfur compounds added to wine as preservatives shows competitive effect to selenium [55].

3.5. Lead (Pb)

Pb is toxic elements, taken from food and drinking water. Pb may accumulate in selected organs, such as blood, liver, kidney, brain and bone [56]. Toxic effects of Pb reveal in disorders of the circulatory system in the form of inhibition of synthesis of hemoglobin [57]. In addition to inhibition of enzymes involved in heme synthesis, Pb compounds may impair the functions of central and peripheral nervous system. With chronic exposure, there is also damage kidneys and liver [58]. Pb is considered as a potential immunotoxic factor. It exerts a direct toxic effect on cells of the immune system or modulate the immune response to antigens and mitogens, and also causes contact allergy and induces autoimmune disease [59].

There were no significant differences in the concentration of Pb in blood and aortic wall of patients with AAA (27.96 ± 20.3 µg/L, 162.65 ± 157.2 ng/g, respectively) compared to controls (33.25 ± 11.1 µg/L and 137.16 ± 134.2 ng/g, respectively) - Table 5. The average concentration of Pb in the parietal thrombus was 7.97 9.6 ng/g. We found a significantly higher ($p < 0.05$) concentration of Pb in aortic wall samples of smoking than non-smoking patients [51].

In patients with CA the blood Pb concentration (48.98 ± 37.4 µg/L) was significantly higher ($p < 0.028$) compared to healthy people (29.63 ± 22.8 µg/L) - Table 5 [60].

Approximately 80% of Pb absorbs to the body through food. The source of Pb in the diet is mostly plant food: leafy and root vegetables, potatoes, cereals, legumes, cucurbits and tomatoes. Offal, meat and fish also may be contaminated with Pb compounds and processes, and packaging add to the contents of Pb in food [56].

The concentration of Pb can increase the frequent consumption of wholegrain products, and cooked vegetables, but consumption of grits, rice and honey may have positively influence on Pb status [51,60].

3.6. Cadmium (Cd)

Cd, like Pb, is also a toxic element. Interaction of Cd with elements such as Zn, Cu, Fe, Mg, Ca, Se, which are essential for the body, causes morphological and functional changes in specific organs. Cd impairs carbohydrate metabolism, insulin secretion, inhibits the activity of oxidases and induces lipid peroxidation. Chronic exposure to Cd deteriorates kidney function, demineralization of bone, nervous system disorders, immune, and hyperglycemia [59,61,62]. Prolonged exposure to Cd can cause cardiovascular diseases. It is known that Cd can affect the formation of hypertension, which is probably caused by insufficient oxygen renin release from the kidney, which accumulate large amounts of metallothionein [63].

Type of aneurysm	Concentration of Pb (average ± SD)		p
AAA	Blood (µg/L)		$p_{1/2} = 0.327$
	1. Control group (n =22)	2. Examined group (n =49)	
	33.25 ± 11.1	27.96 ± 20.3	
	Aortic wall (ng/g)		$p_{3/4} = 0.562$
	3. Without aneurysm (n =17)	4. With aneurysm (n =40)	
	137.16 ± 134.2	162.65 ± 157.2	
CA	Blood (µg/L)		$p_{5/6} < 0.03$
	5. Control group (n =22)	6. Examined group (n =64)	
	29.63 ± 22.75	48.98 ± 37.36 ↑	

SD – standard deviation, p – significance level, n – number of samples

Table 5. Concentration of Pb in patients with abdominal aortic aneurysm (AAA), cerebral aneurysm (CA) and in the control groups.

The average blood Cd concentrations in AAA and CA patients were similar to the control groups. There was also no significant differences in content of Cd between aortic wall with aneurysm and normal aorta - Table 6 [60,64]. Cigarette smoking did not influence on content of Cd in examined patients.

Food is one of the sources of exposure to Cd, in addition to environmental and occupational exposure. High content of Cd may contain offal, fish and seafood and vegetable products from the areas contaminated with this element, such as leafy and root vegetables and mushrooms [56].

The frequent consumption of boiled and raw vegetables, and meat products contributed to the increase concentration of Cd, while frequent consumption of grits and rice decreased its level in the patients with aneurysms. Various species of grits and rice, especially brown rice, due to its high content of essential minerals can protect against the accumulation of toxic elements in the body [60,64].

Type of aneurysm	Concentration of Cd (average ± SD)		p
AAA	Blood ($\mu g/L$)		$p_{1/2} = 0.748$
	1. Control group (n = 20)	2. Examined group (n = 42)	
	2.60 ± 2.42	3.22 ± 2.27	
	Aortic wall (ng/g)		$p_{3/4} = 0.824$
	3. Without aneurysm (n = 6)	4. With aneurysm (n = 42)	
	75.47 ± 27.27	72.32 ± 32.69	
CA	Blood ($\mu g/L$)		$p_{5/6} = 0.342$
	5. Control group (n = 22)	6. Examined group (n = 64)	
	1.652 ± 1.70	1.252 ± 1.14	

SD – standard deviation, p – significance level, n – number of samples

Table 6. Concentration of Cd in patients with abdominal aortic aneurysm (AAA), cerebral aneurysm (CA) and in the control groups.

4. Conclusions

Serum Zn concentration in patients with AAA and CA is significantly decreased. In turn, serum concentration of Cu in patients with AAA is increased, but decreased in the case of CA. On the other hand, serum concentration of Se in patients with AAA is lower when compared to healthy people, but does not change in the CA. The content of Mg is decreased only in the aortic wall with aneurysm, but its concentration in serum does not change in both types of aneurysms. The concentration of Pb is only increased in the blood of people with CA, while the concentration of Cd in the blood is comparable to healthy people in both types of aneurysms.

Dietary habits (frequency of consumption of each group of food products) may affect directly or indirectly on the content of the Mg, Cu, Zn, Se, Pb and Cd in people with AAA and CA.

Our results may help to explain the role of mineral components in case of aneurysms and be important in the prevention of this diseases.

Author details

Katarzyna Socha* and Maria H. Borawska
Department of Bromatology, Medical University of Bialystok, Poland

---

* Corresponding Author

Acknowledgement

We wish to thank our colleagues: Prof. Marek Gacko, Dr Andrzej Guzowski from Department of Vascular Surgery and Transplantology, Medical University of Bialystok and Prof. Zenon Mariak, Dr hab. Jan Kochanowicz from Department of Neurosurgery, Medical University of Bialystok; for cooperation and clinical consultations.

5. References

[1]   de Figueiredo Borges L, Martelli H, Fabre M, Touat Z, Jondeau G, Michel JB (2010) Histopathology of an Iliac Aneurysm in a Case of Menkes Disease. Pediatr. dev. pathol. 13 (3): 247-251.

[2]   Gacko M, Głowiński S, Worowska A (1999) Zawartość Cynku, Magnezu, Manganu, Miedzi i Żelaza w Ścianie Tętniaka Aorty (in Polish). Biul. magnezol. 4 (2): 322-324.

[3]   Iskra M, Majewski W, Piorunska-Stolzmann M (2002) Modifications of Magnesium and Copper Concentrations in Serum and Arterial Wall of Patients with Vascular Diseases Related to Ageing, Atherosclerosis and Aortic Aneurysm. Magnes. res. 15 (3-4): 279-285.

[4]   Iskra M, Patelski J, Majewski W (1997) Relationship of Calcium, Magnesium, Zinc and Copper Concentrations in the Arterial Wall and Serum in Atherosclerosis Obliterans and Aneurysm. J. trace elem. med. biol. 11 (4): 248-252.

[5]   Koksal C, Ercan M, Bozkurt AK, Cortelekoglu T, Konukoglu D (2007) Abdominal Aortic Aneurysm or Aortic Occlusive Disease: Role of Trace Element Imbalance. Angiology 58 (2): 191-195.

[6]   Gopal K, Kumar K, Nandini R, Jahan P, Kumar MJ (2010) High Fat Diet Containing Cholesterol Induce Aortic Aneurysm Through Recruitment and Proliferation of Circulating Agranulocytes in apoE Knock Out Mice Model. J. thromb. thrombolysis . 30 (2): 154-163.

[7]   Kent KC, Zwolak RM, Egorova NN, Riles TS, Manganaro A, Moskowitz AJ, Gelijns AC, Greco G (2010) Analysis of Risk Factors for Abdominal Aortic Aneurysm in a Cohort of More Than 3 Million Individuals. J. vasc. surg. 52 (3): 539-548.

[8]   Shiue I, Arima H, Hankey GJ, Anderson CS (2011) Dietary Intake of Key Nutrients and Subarachnoid Hemorrhage: a Population-based Case-control Study in Australasia. Cerebrovasc. dis. 31(5): 464-470.

[9]   Wong DR, Willett WC, Rimm EB (2007) Smoking, Hypertension, Alcohol Consumption, and Risk of Abdominal Aortic Aneurysm in Men. Am. j. epidemiol. 165 (7): 838-845.

[10] Sygnowska E, Waśkiewicz A, Pardo B (1997) Zmiany Zwyczajowego Sposobu Żywienia Populacji Warszawy Objętej Programem Pol-MONICA w latach 1984-93 (in Polish). Żyw. człow. metab. 24: 234-248.

[11] Classen HG, Grimm P (1992) Pharmacokinetics of Magnesium Salts. Methods find. exp. clin. 14 (4): 261-268.

[12] Dai Q, Motley SS, Smith JA Jr, Concepcion R, Barocas D, Byerly S, Fowke JH (2011) Blood Magnesium, and the Interaction with Calcium, on the Risk of High-grade Prostate Cancer. PLoS One 6(4): e18237.

[13] Altura BT, Brust M, Bloom S, Barmour RL, Stempak JG, Altura BM (1990) Magnesium Dietary Intake Modulates Blood Lipid Levels and Artherogenesis. Proc. natl. acad sci. USA 87: 1840-1844.

[14] Gacko M (2000) Eksperymentalny Tętniak Aorty (in Polish). Post. hig. med. dośw. 54 (5): 699-722.

[15] Socha K, Borawska M, Gacko M, Guzowski A, Markiewicz R (2006) Dieta a Zawartość Magnezu w Surowicy, Ścianie i Skrzeplinie Przyściennej Tętniaka Aorty Brzusznej (in Polish). Bromat. chem. toksykol. 39: 655-658.

[16] Socha K, Borawska MH, Mariak Z, Kochanowicz J, Soroczyńska J (2009) Dieta a Zawartość Magnezu w Surowicy Pacjentów z Tętniakiem Mózgu (in Polish). Bromat. chem. toksykol. 42: 666-671.

[17] Ziemlański Ś (2001) Normy Żywienia Człowieka. Fizjologiczne Podstawy (in Polish). Warsaw: PZWL. pp. 349-362.

[18] Borawska MH, Czyżewska E, Łazarczyk B, Socha K (2005) Wpływ Nawyków Żywieniowych na Zawartość Magnezu u Ludzi z Nowotworami Krtani (in Polish). Bromat. chem. toksykol. 38: 639-642.

[19] Sobol G, Pyda E, Darmolińska B, Mizia A (2000) Biologiczna Rola Cynku i Miedzi i Ich Znaczenie dla Przebiegu Procesu Zapalnego (in Polish). Przeg. pediat. 30 (1): 7-9.

[20] Grant ME, Steven FS, Jakson DS (1971) Carbohydrate Content of Insoluble Elastins Prepared from Adult Bovine and Calf Ligamentum Nuchae and Tropoelastin Isolated from Copper-deficient Porcine Aorta. Biochem j. 121: 197-202.

[21] Kang YJ (2011) Copper and Homocysteine in Cardiovascular Diseases. Pharmacol. ther. 129(3): 321-31.

[22] López B, González A, Hermida N, Valencia F, de Teresa E, Díez J (2010) Role of Lysyl Oxidase in Myocardial Fibrosis: from Basic Science to Clinical Aspects. Am. j. physiol. heart circ. physiol. 299 (1): H1-9.

[23] Lamb DJ, Leake DS (1994) Acidic pH Enables Ceruloplasmin to Catalyse the Modification of Low Density Lipoprotein. FEBS lett. 338: 122-126.

[24] Nasulewicz A, Opolski A (2002) Rola Miedzi w Procesie Angiogenezy Nowotworowej – Implikacje Kliniczne (in Polish) Post. hig. med. dośw. 6: 691-705.

[25] Hukałowicz K, Borawska M, Gacko M, Guzowski A, Czyżewska E (2004) The Contents of Copper in Serum, Arterial Wall and Parietal Thrombus of Patients with Aortic Abdominal Aneurysm. Metal ions biol. med., 8: 456-459.

[26] Trumbo P, Yates AA, Schlicker S, Poos M (2001) Dietary Reference Intakes: Vitamin A, Vitamin K, Arsenic, Boron, Chromium, Copper, Iodine, Iron, Manganese, Molybdenum, Nickel, Silicon, Vanadium, and Zinc. J. am. diet. assoc. 101 (3): 294-301.

[27] Markiewicz R, Borawska MH, Socha K, Roszkowska M (2006) Content of Selenium and Lead in Some Tissues of Animals from Podlasie as an Indicator of Environmental Conditions. Pol. j. environ. stud. 15 (2a): 135-138.

[28] Nogowska M, Jelińska A, Muszalska I, Stanisz B (2000) Funkcje Biologiczne Makro- i Mikroelementów (in Polish). Farm. pol. 56 (21): 995-1004.

[29] Prasad AS (1983) Zinc Deficiency in Human Subjects. Prog. clin. biol. res. 129: 1-33.

[30] Bao B, Prasad AS, Beck FW. Fitzgerald JT, Snell D, Bao GW, Singh T, Cardozo LJ (2010) Zinc Decreases C-reactive Protein, Lipid Peroxidation, and Inflammatory Cytokines in Elderly Subjects: a Potential Implication of Zinc as an Atheroprotective Agent. Am. j. clin. nutr. 91 (6): 1634-1641.

[31] Kuliczkowski W, Jołda-Mydłowska B, Kobusiak-Prokopowicz M, Antonowicz-Juchniewicz J, Kosmala W (2004) Wpływ Jonów Wybranych Metali Ciężkich na Czynność Śródbłonka u Pacjentów z Chorobą Niedokrwienną Serca (in Polish). Pol. arch. med. wewn. 111 (6): 682-683.

[32] Puzanowska-Tarasiewicz H, Kuźmicka L, Tarasiewicz M (2009) Funkcje Biologiczne Wybranych Pierwiastków. III. Cynk – Składnik i Aktywator enzymów (in Polish). Pol. merk. lek. 161 (27): 419-421.

[33] Panek B, Gacko M, Pałka J (2004) Metalloproteinases, Insulin-like Growth Factor-I and its Binding Proteins in Aortic Aneurysm. Int. j. exp. pathol. 85 (3): 159-164.

[34] Prasad AS, Beck FW, Doerr TD, Shamsa FH, Penny HS, Marks SC, Kaplan J, Kucuk O, Mathog RH (1998) Nutritional and Zinc Status of Head and Neck Cancer Patients: an Interpretive Review. J. am. coll. nutr. 17 (5): 409-418.

[35] Prasad AS, Beck FW, Snell DC, Kucuk O (2009) Zinc in Cancer Prevention. Nutr. cancer.61 (6): 879-887.

[36] Milne D, Canfield W. Mahalko J (1984) Effect of Oral Folic Acid Supplements on Zinc, Copper and Iron Absorption and Excretion. Am. j. clin. nutr. 39: 535-539.

[37] Socha K, Borawska M, Gacko M, Guzowski A, Markiewicz R (2005) Dieta a Zawartość Cynku w Surowicy Krwi, Subkomórkowej Ścianie i Skrzeplinie Przyściennej Tętniaka Aorty (in Polish). Żyw. człow. metab. 32: 380-384.

[38] Socha K, Borawska MH, Mariak Z, Kochanowicz J, Markiewicz R (2009) Diet and Content of Zinc in Serum of Patients with Brain Aneurysm. Fresenius environ. bull. 18, 10a: 1932-1936.

[39] Koźlicka I, Przysławski J (2007) Wpływ Cynku na Występowanie i Przebieg Procesów Chorobowych u Osób Dorosłych (in Polish). Roczn. PZH 58 (3): 557-562.

[40] Schlegel-Zawadzka M (2001) Cynk: Źródła, Biodostępność, Metabolizm, Preparaty cynku. In: Nowak G, editor. Cynk w Fizjologii oraz w Patologii i Terapii Depresji (in Polish). Krakow: Instytut Farmakologii PAN. pp. 2007-2026.

[41] Wąsowicz W, Gromadzińska J, Rydzyński K, Tomczak J (2003) Selenium Status of Low - Selenium Area Residents: Polish Experience. Toxicol. lett. 137: 95-101.

[42] Zachara BA, Pawluk H, Bloch-Bogusławska E, Śliwka KM, Korenkiewicz-Skok Z, Ryć K (2001) Tissue Level, Distribution, and Total Body Selenium Content in Healthy and Diseased Humans in Poland. Arch. environ. health. 56 (5): 461-466.

[43] Holben DH, Smith AM (1999) The Diverse Role of Selenium within Selenoproteins. J. am. diet. assoc. 99 (7): 836-843.

[44] Wesołowski M, Ulewicz B (2000) Selen – Pierwiastek Śladowy Niezbędny dla Człowieka – Występowanie, Znaczenie Biologiczne i Toksyczność (in Polish). Farm. pol. 56 (21): 1004-1019.

[45] El-Bayoumy K (1994) Evaluation of Chemopreventive Agents Breast Cancer and Proposed Strategies for Future Clinical Intervention Trials. Carcinogenesis 15: 2395-2420.

[46] Gromadzińska J, Reszka E, Bruzelius K, Wąsowicz W, Akesson B (2008) Selenium and Cancer: Biomarkers of Selenium Status and Molecular Action of Selenium Supplements. Eur. j. nutr. 47 (2): 29-50.

[47] Jabłońska E, Gromadzińska J, Reszka E, Wąsowicz W, Sobala W, Szeszenia-Dąbrowska N, Boffetta P (2009) Association Between GPx1 Pro198Leu Polymorphism, GPx1 Activity and Plasma Selenium Concentration in Humans. Eur. j. nutr. 48: 383-386.

[48] Reid ME, Duffield-Lillico AJ, Garland L, Turnbull BW, Clark LC, Marshall JR (2002) Selenium Supplementation and Lung Cancer Incidence: an Update of the Nutritional Prevention of Cancer Trial. Cancer epidemiol. biomarkers prev. 11: 1285-1291.

[49] Benton D (2002) Selenium Intake, Mood and Other Aspects of Psychological Functioning. Nutr. neurosci. 5 (6): 363-374.

[50] Neumeister B, Besenthal I, Liebich H (2001) Diagnostyka laboratoryjna (in Polish). Wrocław: Urban & Partner. pp. 212-213.

[51] Socha K, Borawska MH, Gacko M, Guzowski A (2011) Diet and the Content of Selenium and Lead in Patients with Abdominal Aortic Aneurysm. VASA – European journal of vascular medicine 40 (5): 381-389.

[52] Borawska MH, Socha K, Konopka M, Mariak Z, Kochanowicz J (2010) Environmental Conditions and Selenium Status among Patients with Cerebral Aneurysms. Fresenius environ. bull. 19, 2a: 368-371.

[53] Ulewicz-Magulska B, Wesołowski M (2007) Selen jako Naturalny Składnik Mineralny Produktów Żywnościowych Pochodzenia Roślinnego (in Polish). Farm. pol. 63 (19): 869-876.

[54] Markiewicz R, Borawska MH (2005) Mięso jako Źródło Selenu w Diecie Mieszkańców Podlasia (in Polish). Bromat. chem. toksykol. 38: 249-252.

[55] Taylor D, Dalton C, Hall A, Woodroofe MN, Gardiner PH (2009) Recent Developments in Selenium Research. Br. j. biomed. sci. 66 (2): 107-116.

[56] Nabrzyski M (1998) Toksykologiczna ocena wybranych metali śladowych w żywności. In: Problemy jakości analizy śladowej w badaniach środowiska przyrodniczego (in Polish). Warsaw: Wydawnictwo Edukacyjne Zofii Dobkowskiej. pp. 13-40.

[57] Rogival D, Scheirs J, De Coen W, Verhagen R, Blust R (2006) Metal Blood Levels and Hematological Characteristics in Wood Mice (Apodemus Sylvaticus L.) Along a Metal Pollution Gradient. Environ. toxicol. chem. 25: 149-57.

[58] Seńczuk W (1999) Toksykologia (in Polish), Warsaw: PZWL. pp. 490-498.

[59] Zellikeff JT, Smiałowicz R, Bigazzi PE, Goyer RA (1994) Immunomodulation by Metals. Fundam. appl. toxicol. 22: 1-7.

[60] Socha K, Borawska MH, Mariak Z, Kochanowicz J, Markiewicz R, Bącławek E (2009) Dietary Habits and the Content of Lead and Cadmium in the Blood of Patients with Brain Aneurysms. Żyw. człow. metab. 36: 461-467.

[61] Brzóska MM, Jurczuk M, Moniuszko-Jakoniuk J (1997) Interakcje Kadmu z Wybranymi Biopierwiastkami (in Polish). Terapia 5: 28-30.

[62] Merali Z, Kacew S, Sibghal RL (1975) Response of Hepatic Carbohydrate and cAMP Metabolism to Cadmium Treatment in Rats. Can. j. physiol. pharmacol. 53: 174-184.

[63] Markiewicz J (1989) Wybrane Metale Ciężkie w Środowisku Człowieka (Rtęć, Ołów, Kadm). In: Gumińska M, editor. Ekologiczne Zagrożenia Zdrowia Człowieka (in Polish). Kraków: Nauka dla wszystkich, PAN. pp. 61-78.

[64] Socha K, Borawska MH, Gacko M, Guzowski A, Markiewicz R (2005) Dieta a Zawartość Kadmu w Krwi, Subkomórkowej Ścianie i Skrzeplinie Przyściennej Tętniaka Aorty Brzusznej (in Polish). Bromat. chem. toksykol. 38: 51-55.

Chapter 4

The Role of Metalloproteinases in the Development of Aneurysm

Krzysztof Siemianowicz

Additional information is available at the end of the chapter

1. Introduction

Matrix metalloproteinases (MMPs) were first described by Gross fifty years ago. They are a family of zinc-dependent endopeptidases. They comprise a group of 25 enzymes. Metalloproteinases were first described as proteases degrading extracellular matrix (ECM) proteins such as collagens, elastin, proteoglycans and laminins, hence they were named matrix meatalloproteinases. MMPs were divided according to their substrate specificity into collagenases, gelatinases, stromolysins and matrilysins. This classification was later replaced by numbering the enzymes according to the chronology of their identification. Metalloproteinases are also called metalloproteases.

Four metalloproteases (MMP-14, MMP-15, MMP-16 and MMP-24) have a transmembrane and cytosolic domains. They constitute a subgroup of membrane-type metalloproteases (MT-MMPs) [1, 2].

2. Physiological role of metalloproteinases

MMP-1 (collagenase 1) hydrolyzes collagen types I, II, III, VII, VIII, X and XI, as well as gelatin, fibronectin, vitronectin, laminin, tenascin, aggrecan, links protein, myelin basic protein and versican. MMP-2 (gellatinase) degrades collagen types I, II, III, IV, V, VII, X and XI, gelatin, elastin, fibronectin, vitronectin, laminin, entactin, tenascin, SPARC and aggrecan, links protein, galectin-3, versican, decanin and myelin basic protein. One of the most important differences between theses two metalloproteinases is the possibility of the hydrolysis of elastin and collagen type IV by MMP-2, but not by MMP-1. Researches have also focused their interest on MMP-9 which can degrade collagen types IV, V, VII, X and XIV, fibronectin, laminin, nidogen, proteoglycan link protein and versican.

For a long time metalloproteinases have been vied solely as enzymes of matrix proteins breakdown. Results of researches performed in recent years indicate that there is a group of non-matrix proteins which can be substrates for various MMPs. Metalloproteinases are involved in the activation of latent forms of effective proteins. For example, MMP-2, MMP-3 and MMP-9 can activate interleukin 1β (IL-1β). They can also act on active cytokines, IL-1β undergoes subsequent degradation catalyzed by MMP-3. Metalloproteinases can alter cell surface proteins such as receptors and act on microbial peptides.

Metalloproteinases are not indiscriminately released by cells. They are secreted to or anchored to cell membrane. MT-MMPs have a specific transmembrane domain placing them in a certain position. Other metalloproteinases can be bound by specific cell-MMP interactions. This phenomenon allows an exact localization of their proteolytic activity [1,2].

3. Activation of metalloproteinases

Metalloproteinases are encoded as inactive proenzymes, zymogens. They undergo proteolytic activation. This process can take place either intracellulary or extracellulary. One third of MMPs are activated by intracellular serin protease, furin. This process takes place in trans-Golgi network. A number of MMPs has a cleavage site for other metalloproteinases. MMP-3 activates proMMP-1 and pro-MMP-7. Some metalloproteinases have been described to be activated by kallikrein or plasmin.

In vivo studies indicate that reactive oxygen species (ROS) generated by neutrophils can both activate and subsequently inactivate MMPs. Hypochlorus acid (HClO) generated by neutrophil myeloperoxidase and hydroxyl radicals can activate proMMP-1, proMMP-7 and proMMP-9, whereas peroxynitrate can activate proenzymes of MMP-1, MMP-2 and MMP-9. This process enables a control of burst of proteolytic activity within an inflammatory setting.

Like some other proteases, activity of MMPs is controlled also by two other mechanisms, regulation of gene expression and specific inhibitors. MMP-2 is constitutively expressed and regulation of its activity occurs by either activation or inhibition. Expression of a number of metalloproteinases is up-regulated during various pathological conditions. Among them inflammation is the most studied setting. MMPs are inhibited by α-2 macroglobulin and tissue inhibitors of metalloproteinases (TIMPs). There are four TIMPs. Their secretion is also regulated and represents another point in a network of control of the activity of metalloproteinases. TIMP-3 is primarily bond to ECM and allows a regulation of MMPs' activity in the very site of their action. The network of the control of the activity of metalloproteinases is complex and very precise. Sometimes TIMP interacts with proMMP and inactivate other MMP, e.g. a complex of TIMP-1 and proMMP-9 inactivates MMP-3.

Protection from MMP degradation represents the next step in this sophisticated network of diverse interactions. Neutrophil gelatinase-associated lipocalin (NGAL) bounds to MMP-9 protecting this metalloproteinase from its degradation [1,2].

4. Localisation of metalloproteinases in a vascular wall

Metalloproteinases can be detected in all three layers of a vascular wall. Endothelium can produce MMP-1 and MMP-2. Smooth muscle cells (SMC) of both intima and media are the next source of MMPs. They can secrete MMP-2 and MMP-9. SMC can also produce TIMP-1 and TIMP-2. Adventitia is the layer where MMP-9 can be synthesized. Apart from these most studied metalloproteinases some other MMPs can be detected in a vascular wall: MT1-MMP, MMP-3, MMP-8, MMP-10, MMP-12 and MMP-13. Metalloproteinases are found not only in a wall of arterial wall, but in veins as well.

The balance between the expression of MMPs and TIMPs plays a vital role in preserving the proper and health state of the vascular wall. This equilibrium between activation and inactivation of MMPs is a part of a balance between synthesis and degradation of collagen and elastin, two proteins which have various properties and functions in the arterial wall. Both proteins are crucial for a proper function of the arterial wall. An interruption of these two balances may lead to a development of various vascular pathologies including atherosclerosis, formation of aneurysm and inflammation [3-5].

5. Metalloproteinases and aneurysms

The most studied aneurysm is abdominal aortic aneurysm (AAA), far less research has been focused on aneurysms of cerebral arteries and thoracic aortic aneurysm. All aneurysms are characterized by the destruction of the structural integrity of the extracellular matrix proteins, mainly collagens and elastin. MMPs involved in this pathology can origin both from the cells that physiologically constitute the arterial wall and are stimulated to secrete MMPs, i.e. endothelium, SMC and cells that infiltrate the arterial wall in a response to various stimuli [1, 3, 6-9].

Many scientists points out that cells constituting an inflammatory infiltrate are the major source of metalloproteinases involved in the development of aneurysms. Studies of samples derived from patients undergoing surgery for AAA demonstrated that macropgages from the inflammatory infiltrate can express MMP-1, MMP-2, MMP-3, MMP-9 and MT-1MMP. Metalloproteinase-2 was often detected in cells physiologically constituting the arterial wall, but was absent in macrophages within aneurysms. The pathogenesis of AAA and aneurysms of cerebral arteries differs as these vessels present different types of arteries and there are some differences in the physical characteristic of blood flow in them. Recent experimental studies carried on animals confirmed the role of macrophage infiltration in the formation of intracranial aneurysms. A degranulation of mast cells induces the expression and activation of MMP-2 and MMP-9. Inhibitors of mast cell degranulation inhibited the development of cerebral aneurysms in experimental rats [10, 11].

Human studies confirmed that the expression of metalloproteinases within the AAA is greater than in other sites, remote from the dissection. Nishimura *et al.* observed a different profile of MMP activation in small size abdominal aortic aneurysms, less than 45 mm and large size AAA with diameter exceeding 45 mm. In small size AAA MMP-2 and MMP-9 presented greater gene expression whereas in large size AAA membrane type-1 metalloproteinase and MMP-9 had greater expression. The same study demonstrated also differences in the distribution of the metalloproteinases in the arterial wall. MMP-2 was detected mainly in the intima, whereas MMP-9 was present both in intima and adventitia.

Nishimura *et al.* also observed a significant correlation of the expression of MMP-2 and MMP-9 and between each of these metalloproteinases and TIMP-1 [6].

The degeneration of collagen and elastin leading to the development of aneurysms is a multifactorial process. Various factors may take part in the stimulation of both cells constituting the arterial wall and cells infiltrating it to produce MMPs. Aortic wall is subjected to cyclic stretching because of pulsative blood flow which is a normal physiological condition. AAA is often accompanied by an intraluminal thrombus. It causes that some cells within the aneurysm may be subjected to hypoxia. Experimental study of Oya *et al.* revealed that macrophages cultured in conditions subjected to cyclic stretching under normoxia and hypoxia which simulated the pulsative blood flow and hypoxia due to thrombus presented an increased MMP-9 production. These macrophages produced interleukin-8 (IL-8) and tumor necrosis factor-α (TNF-α) leading to increased apoptosis of vascular smooth muscle cells. Hypoxia was also demonstrated to augment the expression of MMP-1, MT-1 MMP, MMP-2, MMP-7 and MMP-9 in SMC derived from human aorta [12, 13].

Nowadays many scientists focus their research on finding new factors which may augment the secretion of metalloproteinases by the cells present in aneurysms. Experimental studies confirmed that stenosis resulting in a turbulent blood flow can be the next factor increasing expression of MMP-2 and MMP-9 within abdominal aortic aneurysm. Interesting results were obtained by Stolle *et al.* Mice exposed to cigarette smoke and angiotensin II treatment had increased the incidence of AAA and higher gene expression of MMP-2, MMP-3, MMP-8, MMP-9 and MMP-12 in aorta and increased proteolytic activity of two most investigated metalloproteinaes, MMP-2 and MMP-9. Although each of this two factors alone induced minor changes, their combination accelerated the pathologic process. Exposure of the arterial wall to an increased concentration of angiotensin II represents conditions that may be observed in patients with arterial hypertension. This experiment demonstrates that coexistance of arterial hypertension and smoking augments the risk of a development of aneurysm [14, 15].

Studies of Zhang *et al.* demonstrated that human AAA tissues had elevated levels of advanced glycation end products (AGEs) and their receptor (RAGE). In experimental model this group of researchers observed that AGEs induce the production of MMP-9 by macrophages. An increased serum concentration of AGEs accompanies poorly controlled diabetes mellitus. These results indicate that such patients may be at a greater risk of a development of AAA [16].

Abdominal aortic aneurysm is characterized not only by the destruction of its structural integrity of the extracellular matrix protein and inflammatory infiltrate but also by intensive neovascularisation. These new blood vessels developing inside the arterial wall in a place of growing aneurysm are the next source of metalloproteinases degrading ECM. Immature neovessels express MMP-1, MMP-2, MMP-3, MMP-7, MMP-8, MMP-9 and MMP-12 [8].

Polish scientists have observed that the intraluminal thrombus occurring within AAA may modulate the activity of MMP-8, MMP-9, neutrophil elastase and TIMP-1. Specimens from patients with thin, less than 10 mm, thrombus-covered wall of AAA presented significantly higher activity of 3 evaluated metalloproteinases and lower TIMP-1 concentration than thick, exceeding 25 mm, thrombus-covered wall. The intraluminal thrombus may exert its pathological effect through trapping erythrocyte and neutrophils and monocytes. The exact mechanism of activation of MMP in these conditions has not been fully elucidated. Scientists consider various factors activating metalloproteinases, such as hypoxia caused by reduced blood flow or oxidative stress in trapped blood cells. This aspect needs further evaluation [17].

Japanese researchers compared the activity of MMP-2 and MMP-9 in ruptured and unruptured middle cerebral artery dissections obtained during neurosurgery in the same patient. Both metalloproteinases presented greater expression in the ruptured dissection [9].

6. Possible diagnostic markers

The results of scientific researches discussed so far concern the evaluation of either expression or activity of MMPs in the tissue obtained from aneurysms in humans or experimental animals. These measurements have the scientific importance but cannot serve as a diagnostic marker. A growing interest is focused on finding circulating predictors of risk of the development of aneurysm or plasma markers of existing, yet undiagnosed aneurysm. Plasma levels of MMPs are of great interest. MMP-2 and MMP-9 are the candidates for such markers. Polish researchers observed significantly higher plasma concentration of MMP-9 in patients with AAA and thin intraluminal thrombus than in patients with abdominal aortic aneurysm and thick thrombus. Hellenthal *et al.* points out that plasma level of MMP-9 may serve as a marker discriminating patients with and without endoleak within AAA [18-20].

Several polymorphisms of metalloproteinases have been discovered. Their role in the development of AAA is being studied. The polymorphisms of MMP-2 (1306C/T), MMP-3 (5A/6A) and MMP-13 (77A/G) may contribute to the pathogenesis of AAA. The studies of circulating markers of aneurysms give promising results but further research is still required [21].

7. Visualisation of metalloproteinases in aneurysm

Several studies have been aimed at imaging of matrix metalloproteinases and quantifying the inflammatory process that drives abdominal aortic aneurysm development. American scientists developed the MMP-activated probe, MMP Sense 18-20 (VisEn Medical, Woburn, USA) that was used for the *in vivo* and *ex vivo* macroscopic scale imaging. This method based on fluorochromes may be used intravascularly. A new magnetic resonance imaging contrast agent, P947, has been tested for its capabilities of targeting MMPs *in vivo* in expanding experimental AAA. This method allows the detection of MMP activity within the inflammatory infiltrate within AAA and may become a potential non-invasive method to detect AAA at a high risk of rupture [22, 23].

8. Possibilities of pharmacological modulation of metalloproteinases activity

Patients with a high activity of MMPs within the aneurysm are at increased risk of its rupture leading to serious clinical consequences including death. It is of a great importance to find agents which can inhibit MMPs activity and reduce this risk.

Doxycycline, a tetracycline antibiotic, is a known inhibitor of metalloproteinases activity with a growing body of evidence of its beneficial effects observed in animal studies. However data from human studies comprising 6 controlled trials and 2 cohort studies gave conflicting results. The safety of long term use of doxycycline needs evaluation [24].

Statins are a well known group of drugs lowering plasma cholesterol level used to reduce the risk of a coronary heart disease. They have a pleiotropic mode of action reducing the progress of atherosclerosis. Experimental studies indicate that simvastatin can reduce the activity of MMP-2 and MMP-9 in AAA and suppress the development and expansion of abdominal aortic aneurysm. A study performed on samples derived from patients receiving atorvastatin and undergoing surgical treatment for AAA gave promising results demonstrating a significantly reduced activity of MMP-13. Another study with short term, 4 weeks, administration of atorvastatin preceding the operation did not show any differences in the activity of MMP-2, MMP-8, MMP-9, TIMP-1 or TIMP-2. These data indicate that statins may require a long term use to develop their beneficial influence on MMPs' activity [25-27].

Drugs which are administered for a long time focus the scientists' interest. Anti-hypertensive drugs have been studied in this aspect. Calcium channel blocker, azelnidipine, decreased the activity of MMP-2 and MMP-9. The similar influence of angiotensin II receptor blockers, olmesartan and losartan, was observed. The latter was also shown to act synergistically with doxycycline. Perindopril, an angiotensin converting enzyme inhibitor, is known as an anti-hypertensive agent with an ability to affect vascular wall remodeling. In an experimental study perindopril significantly reduced the activity of MMP-2 and MMP-9. In animal studies the activity of MMP-2 and MMP-9 were also decreased by edaravone, a scavenger of reactive oxygen species, resveratrol, a plant derived polyphenolic compound. Two inhibitors of cyclic adenosine monophosphate phosphodiesterase (PDE) were also shown to inhibit the activity of metalloproteinases. Cilostazol, the inhibitor of PDE-3 decreased the activity of MMP-2 and MMP-9, whereas ibudilast, which predominantly blocked PDE-4, decreased the expression of MMP-9 [28-37].

Although the experimental studies indicate that various drugs can reduce the expression and activity of metalloproteinases, their potential use in humans to protect from AAA or inhibit its development requires further studies. Their efficacy and safety of a long term administration must be proven.

Author details

Krzysztof Siemianowicz
Medical University of Silesia, Department of Biochemistry, Poland

9. References

[1] Pearce W.H. & Shively V.P. (2006). Abdominal aortic aneurysm as a complex multifactorial disease. *Annals of New York Academy of Sciences* (1085): 117-132

[2] Ra H-J. & Parks W.C. (2007). Control of matrix metalloproteinase catalytic activity. *Matrix Biology* (26): 587-596

[3] Goodall S. & Crowther M. & Hemingway D.M. &Bell P.R. & Thompson M.M. (2001). Ubiquitous elevation of matrix metalloproteinase-2 expression in the vasculature of patients with abdominal aneurysms. *Circulation* (104): 304-309

[4] Ishii T. & Asuwa N. (2000). Collagen and elastin degradation by matrix metalloproteinases and tissue inhibitors of matrix metalloproteinases in aortic dissection. *Human Pathology* (31): 640-646

[5] Siemianowicz K. & Gminski J. & Goss M. & Francuz T. & Likus W. & Jurczak T. & Garczorz W. (2010). Influence of elastin-derived peptides on metaloprotease production in endothelial cells. *Experimental and Therapeutical Medicine* (1): 1057-1060

[6] Nishimura K. & Ikebuchi M. & Kanaoka Y. & Ohgi S. & Ueta E. & Nanba E. & Ito H. (2003). Relationship between matrix metalloproteinases and tissue inhibitors of metalloproteinases in the wall of abdominal aortic aneurysms. (2003). *International Journal of Angiology* (22): 229-238

[7] Michel J.B. & Martin-Ventura J.L. & Egido J. & Sakalihasan N. & Treska V. & Lindholt J. & Allaire E. & Thorsteinsdottir U. & Cockerill G. & FAD UE consortium. (2011). Novel aspects of the pathogenesis of aneurysms of the abdominal aorta in humans. *Cardiovascular Research* (90): 18-27

[8] Reeps C. & Pelisek J. & Seidl S. & Schuster T. & Zimmerman A. & Kuehnl A. & Eckstein H.H. (2009). Inflammatory infiltrates and neovessels are relevant sources of MMPs in abdominal aortic aneurysm wall. *Pathobiology* (76): 243-252

[9] Saito A. & Fujimura M. & Inoue T. & Shimizu H. & Tominada T. (2010). Lectin-like oxidized low-density lipoprotein receptor 1 and matrix metalloproteinase expression in ruptured and unruptured multiple dissections of distal middle cerebral artery: case report. *Acta Neurochirurgica* (Wien) (152): 1235-1240

[10] Kanematsu Y. & Kanematsu M. & Kurihara C. & Tada Y. & Tsou T.L. & van Rooijen N. & Lawton M.T. & Young W.L. & Liang E.L. & Nuki Y. & Hashimoto T. (2011). Critical roles of macrophages in the formation of intracranial aneurysm. *Stroke* (42): 173-178

[11] Ishibashi R. & Aoki T. & Nishimura M. & Hashimoto N. & Miyamoto S. (2010). Contribution of mast cells to cerebral aneurysm formation. *Current Neurovascular Research* (7): 113-124

[12] Oya K. & Sakamoto N. & Ohashi T. & Sato M. (2011). Combined stimulation with cyclic stretching and hypoxia increases production of matrix metalloproteinase-9 and cytokines by macrophages. *Biochemical and Biophysical Research Communications* (412): 676-682

[13] Erdozain O.J. & Pegrum S. & Winrow V.R. & Horrocks M. & Stevens C.R. (2010). Hypoxia in abdominal aortic aneurysm supports a role for HIF-1α and Ets-1 as drivers of matrix metalloproteinase upregulation in human aortic smooth muscle cells. *Journal of Vascular Research* (48): 163-170

[14] Mata K.M. & Prudente P.S. & Rocha F.S. & Prado C.M. & Floriano E.M. & Elias J. Jr & Rizzi E. & Gerlach R.F. & Rossi M.A. & Ramos S.G. (2011). Combining two potential causes of metalloproteinase secretion causes abdominal aortic aneurysms in rats: a new experimental model. *International Journal of Experimental Pathology* (92): 26-39

[15] Stolle K. & Berges A. & Lietz M. & Lebrum S. & Wallerath T. (2010). Cigarette smoke enhances abdominal aortic aneurysm formation in angiotensin II-treated apolipoprotein E-defficient mice. (2010). *Toxicology Letters* (199): 403-409

[16] Zhang F. & Banker G. & Liu X. & Suwanabol P.A. & Lengfeld J. & Yamanouchi D. & Kent K.C. & Liu B. (2011). The novel function of advanced glycation end products in regulation of MMP-9 production. *Journal of Surgical Research* (171): 871-876

[17] Wiernicki I. & Stachowska E. & Safranow K. & Cnotliwy M. & Rybicka M. & Kaczmarczyk M. & Gutowski P. (2010). Enhanced matrix-degradating proteolytic activity within the thin thrombus-covered wall of human abdominal aortic aneurysms. *Atherosclerosis* (212): 161-165

[18] Hellenthal F.A. & Ten Bosch J.A. & Pulinx B. & Wodzig W.K. & de Haan M.W. & Prins M.H. & Welten R.J. & Teijink J.A. & Schurink G.W. (2012). Plasma levels of matrix metalloproteinase-9: a possible diagnostic marker of successful endovascular aneurysm repair. *European Journal of Vascular and Endovascular Surgery* (43): 171-172

[19] Wiernicki I. & Millo B. & Safranow K. & Gorecka-Szyld B. & Gutowski P. (2011). MMP-9, homocysteine and CRP circulating levels are associated with intraluminal thrombus thickness of abdominal aortic aneurysms: a new implication of the old biomarkers. *Disease Markers* (31): 67-74

[20] Wen D. & Zhou X.L. & Li J.J. & Hui R.T. (2011). Biomarkers in aortic dissection. *Clinica Chimica Acta* (412): 688-695

[21] Saracini C. & Bolli P. & Sticchi E. & Pratesi G. & Pulli R. & Sofi F. & Pratesi C. & Gensini G.F. Abbate R. & Giusti B. (2012). Polymorphisms of genes involved in extracellular matrix remodeling and abdominal aortic aneurysm. *Vascular Surgery* (55): 171-179

[22] Sheth R.A. & Maricevich M. & Mahmood U. (2010). In vivo optical molecular imaging of matrix metalloproinase activity in abdominal aortic aneurysms correlates with treatment effects on growth rate. *Atherosclerosis* (212): 181-187

[23] Bazeli R. & Coutard M. & Duport B.D. & Lancelot E. & Corot C. & Laissy J.P. & Letourneur D. & Michel J.B. & Serfaty J.M. (2010): In vivo evaluation of a new magnetic

resonance imaging contrast agent (P947) to target matrix metalloproteinases in expanding experimental abdominal aortic aneurysms. *Investigative Radiology* (45): 662-668

[24] Dodd B.R. & Spence R.A. (2011). Doxycycline inhibition of abdominal aortic aneurysm growth: a systemic review of literature. *Current Vascular Pharmacology* (9): 471-478

[25] Mastoraki S.T. & Toumpoulis I.K. & Anagnostopoulos C.E. & Tiniakos D. & Papalois A. & Chamogeorgakis T.P. & Angouras D.C. & Rokkas C.K. (2012). Treatment with simvastatin inhibits the formation of abdominal aortic aneurysms in rabbits. *Annals of Vascular Surgery* (26): 250-258

[26] Schweitzer M. & Mitmaker B. & Obrand D. & Sheiner N. & Abraham C. & Dostanic S. & Meilleur M. & Sugahara T. & Chalifour L.E. (2010). Atorvastatin modulates matrix metalloproteinase expression, activity, and signaling in abdominal aortic aneurysms. *Vascular and Endovascular Surgery* (2010): 116-122

[27] Rahman M.N. & Khan J.A. & Mazari F.A. & Mockford K. & McCollum P.T. & Chetter I.C. (2011). A randomized placebo controlled trial of the effect of preoperative statin use on matrix metalloproteinases and tissue inhibitors of matrix metalloproteinases in areas of low and peak wall stress in patients undergoing elective open repair of abdominal aortic aneurysm. (2011). *Annals of Vascular Surgery* (25): 32-38

[28] Nakamura E. & Akashi H. & Hiromatsu S. & Tanaka A. & Onitsuka S. & Aoyagi S. (2009). Azelnidipine decreases plasma matrix metalloproteinase-9 levels after endovascular abdominal aortic aneurysm repair. *Kurume Medical Journal* (56): 25-32

[29] Yokokura H. & Hiromatsu S. & Akashi H. & Kato S. & Aoyagi S. (2007). Effects of calcium channel blocker azelnidipine on experimental abdominal aortic aneurysms. *Surgery Today* (37): 468-473

[30] Yang H.H. & Kim. J.M. & Chum E. & van Breemen C. & Chung A.W. (2009). Long-term effects of losartan on structure and function of the thoracic aorta in a mouse model of Marfan syndrome. *British Journal of Pharmacology* (158): 1503-1512

[31] Yang H.H. & Kim J.M. & Chum E. & van Breemen C. & Chung A.W. (2010). Effectiveness of combination of losartan potassium and doxycycline versus single-drug treatments in the secondary prevention of thoracic aortic aneurysm in Marfan syndrome. *Journal of Thoracic and Cardiovascular Surgery* (140): 305-312

[32] Alsac J.M. & Journe C. & Louedec L. & Dai J. & Fabiani J.N. & Mitchel J.B. (2011). Downregulation of remodelling enzymatic activity induced by angiotensin-converting enzyme inhibitor (perindopril) reduces the degeneration of experimental abdominal aortic aneurysms in a rat model. *European Journal of Vascular and Endovascular Surgery* (41): 474-480

[33] Hosokawa Y. (2010). Effects of angiotensin receptor blocker and calcium channel blocker on experimental abdominal aortic aneurysms in a hamster model. *Kurume Medical Journal* (57): 1-8

[34] Morimoto K. & Hasegawa T. & Tanaka A. & Wulan B. & Yu J. & Morimoto N. & Okita Y. & Okada K. (2012). Free radical scavenger receptor edaravone inhibits both formation and development of abdominal aortic aneurysm in rats. *Journal of Vascular Surgery* (Epub ahead of print)

[35] Kaneko H. & Anzai T. & Morisawa M. & Nagai T. & Anzai A. & Takahashi T. & Shimoda M. & Sasaki A. & Maekawa Y. & Yoshimura K. & Aoki H. & Tsubota K. & Yoshikawa T. & Okada Y. Ogawa S. & Fukuda K. (2011). Resveratrol prevents the development of abdominal aortic aneurysm through attenuation of inflammation, oxidative stress, and neovascularisation. *Atherosclerosis* (217): 360-367

[36] Zhang Q. & Huang J.H. & Xia R.P. & Duan X.H. & Jiang Y.B. & Jiang Q. & Sun W.J. (2011). Suppresion of experimental abdominal aortic aneurysm in a rat model by phosphodiesterase 3 inhibitor cilostazol. *Journal of Surgical Research* (167): 385-393

[37] Yagi K. & Tada Y. & Kitazato K.T. & Tamura T. & Satomi J. & Nagahiro S. (2010). Ibudilast inhibits cerebral aneurysms by down-regulating inflammation-related molecules in the vascular wall of rats. *Neurosurgery* (66): 551-559

Abdominal Aneurysm

Biomechanical Approach to Improve the Abdominal Aortic Aneurysm (AAA) Rupture Risk Prediction

Guillermo Vilalta, Félix Nieto, Enrique San Norberto,
María Ángeles Pérez, José A. Vilalta and Carlos Vaquero

Additional information is available at the end of the chapter

1. Introduction

It is well known that the human body operates under a continuous interaction of complex processes taking place at multiple dimensional and temporal scales. While biomedical research is slowly elucidating many of these processes, it remains mostly unclear how they interact in the production of the global physiological or pathological conditions we observe [1]. The cardiovascular system in general and the Abdominal Aortic Aneurysms (AAA) in particular is a good example.

Aneurysm is a pathology that can affect most blood vessels, arteries or veins, and it commonly occurs in the cerebral vasculature and the thoracic aorta even if the vast majority of cases occur in the abdominal aorta and are termed AAA.

In its most accepted definition, AAA is a localized, progressive and permanent dilation (usually larger than 3 cm in diameter) of the aortic wall. Under specific conditions mainly associated with an irreversible pathological remodelling of arterial connective tissue, the aneurysm tends to increase in size, with an increased risk of rupture which can cause death. Atherosclerosis is the most common cause of aortic aneurysm. However the causes are usually multifactorial: environmental, genetic, autoimmune or infectious.

AAA has increasingly been recognized as an important health problem in the last decades. The statistics associated with this pathology are the major concern: AAA has been estimated to occur in 3-9% of the population [2], with a mortality rate on rupture between 78-94% [3] producing more than 15,000 deaths annually in the US and 8,000 in England. The mean age of patients with AAA is 67 years and men are affected more than women by a ratio 4:1 with prevalence up to 5% [4].

The majority of studies found in medical literature report this increase in the incidence of aortic aneurismal disease, which is expected in a continuously aging population in developed countries. In spite of significant improvement in surgical procedures and technological advancements in imaging devices in recent years, the associated aneurysm mortality and morbidity rate have also risen concomitantly.

Currently, the lack of an accurate AAA rupture risk index remains an important problem in the clinical management of the disease. The main clinical criteria in deciding on the treatment of AAA patients are: a) the peak transverse diameter and b) the growth rate. If the peak diameter reaches the upper threshold (5-5.5 cm) or the maximum diameter expansion rate is > 0.5 cm/yr for smaller AAAs the patient may be submitted for surgical intervention, also depending on the state of health and willingness of the patients. The main limitation of this practice is that these criteria, although have a significant empirical basis, can be considered insufficient because they have not a physically sound theoretical basis. This statement should not be surprising; approximately 33% of ruptured AAAs have diameters smaller than 50 mm [5] which is indicative of the complex pathogenesis of the disease progression that cannot be capture by traditional indicators.

Due to these observations, recently researches have been focused at improving the knowledge and the understanding of the phenomena associated with the formation and evolution of aneurysm pathology in order to define whether other variables could be predictive of rupture. The literature begins to reflect the existence of a consensus that, rather than empirical criteria, the develop of a biomechanical approach based on a multiscale model can be a significant step for the accurate assessment of the rupture risk.

This chapter examines the basis of the biomechanical approach. The main aim is to support the hypothesis that biomechanical considerations may become into powerful tool for a reliable patient-specific prediction of AAA rupture risk.

2. Biomechanical approach. Method grounds

This new approach has its foundation in the integration, through appropriate relations, of factors from different natures (biological, structural and geometric) and scales (temporal and dimensional) at the molecular, cellular, tissue and organ levels (from bottom level to top level), which allow to describe, from quantitatively point of view, the aneurysm progression and its rupture potential.

These defined relations are known as biomechanical factors or biomechanical determinants (BDs).

The basic premise of the biomechanical approach to estimate the AAA rupture risk, is that this phenomenon follows the principle of material failure, that is, an aneurysm ruptures when the stresses acting on the arterial wall exceeding its failure strength, reflecting the interaction between the arterial wall structural remodelling and the forces generated by blood flow within the AAA.

3. Remodeling history model. Biological Biodeterminants, BBDs

Most investigators would agree that the pathogenesis of the abdominal aortic aneurysm (AAA) is multifactorial. There appear to be environmental, genetic, autoimmune, inflammatory, and structural factors.

The term "atherosclerotic AAA" is misleading because it suggests that atherosclerosis is a necessary cause of AAA disease. While some patients with have atherosclerotic occlusive peripheral vascular disease, others have minimal atherosclerotic disease. For this reason, the Joint Committee of the Society for Vascular Surgery recommending that the term "non-specific AAA" be used since 1991.

The definition of AAA has varied in the literature over the years, but all definitions have in common a specification of the degree of aortic dilatation. So, the definition is a permanent localized dilatation of an artery having at least a 50% increase in diameter compared with the expected normal diameter of the artery or of the diameter of the segment proximal to the dilatation. According to this definition, an infrarenal AAA could then be defined as 3.0 cm if 2.0 cm is the expected maximal diameter of the infrarenalaort in an individual of a specific body scale.

Risk factors

The four principal positive risk factors for AAA are smoking, age, male sex, and family history. While smoking clearly seems to be an environmental factor, issues related to addiction and dose-effect responses are doubtless modified by genetic influences. The three principal negative risk factors for AAA are diabetes, female sex, and African-American descent, all of which are genetically determined.

There is a more complicated relationship between plasma lipid levels and the risk of AAA. Blanchard et al [6], failed to show any correlation between cholesterol levels, low-density lipoprotein (LDL) or high-density lipoprotein (HDL) and aneurysm risk (Blanchard). However, it have been showed an increased risk in patients whose plasma cholesterol was high and a protective effect was seen in patients whose serum HDL was high [7]. Low serum HDL gave an increased risk of AAA [8].

There is some disagreement in the literature regarding the effect of hypertension on aneurysm risk. The American Veterans study represented the largest of its type and showed hypertension to be an independent risk factor. Taking medication for high blood pressure was a risk factor, whereas hypertension itself was significant in women. Tornwall and Blanchard both showed both systolic and diastolic hypertension to be risks [6]. A study of all men born in Malmo in the year 1914 failed to demonstrate hypertension as a risk factor at all [9]. Experimentally, AAAs artificially induced into hypertensive rats were found to grow larger than those in normotensives [10] and the dilatation correlated well with systolic pressure.

Molecular genetics

Epidemiologic review indicates an aneurysm gene expression that is typically delayed until at least the sixth decade. There is strong evidence for inherited predisposition, and possibly an association with generalized arteriomegaly. It have been demonstrated an incidence of 20% aortic aneurysms among first order relatives of aneurysm patients [11]. In [12] was showed genetic linkages, accounting for abdominal aneurysm formation in 50 families, who had clustering of the lesion in two or more first order relatives. Possibly, they possessed a common metabolic disorder affecting the arterial wall.

A retrospective study of hospital patients in Zimbabwe demonstrated a higher incidence of aneurysms among whites than Africans [13]. By using ultrasound screening of first degree relatives demonstrated aortic aneurysms in 20–30% of male siblings over 55 years of age [14]. Case reports of familial aneurysm disease in patients without connective tissue or vascular diseases add validity to the theory of genetic linkage. The occurrence of multiple aneurysms in individuals is consistent with a genetic foundation. Many authors suggest aneurysm disease is a systemic process. Frequently, patients suffer from generalized arteriomegaly; often this is accompanied by multiple aneurysms.

Several cross-linking defects have been associated with aneurysm formation. Tilsonstudied the biochemistry of a collagen component deficiency that predisposes to aneurysms [12]. They evaluated pyridine cross-linkages and found fewer cross-linkages per collagen molecule in human skin samples. This suggests a genetic basis for aneurysm disease. Experiments with sex-linked defects of collagen and elastin demonstrate the blotchy BLO allele. These models exhibit aortic aneurysms and diminished skin tensile strength. The pattern of expression indicates the trait is related to the X chromosome. In [15] it was reviewed the literature and found clear evidence for an independent genetic defect in most AAAs. Their work centered on a genetic analysis of collagen genes. Genetic collagen defects causing architectural defects are established in osteogenesisimperfecta (type I collagen of bone) and chondrodysplasias (type II collagen of cartilage). New evidence implicates mutations in the type III procollagen gene in the pathogenesis of aneurysmal disease. Various mutations have been confirmed in studies of patients with type IV Ehlers–Danlos syndrome (EDS) [16].

Studies of patients with aneurysms clearly demonstrate family linkage, and the data strongly suggest a genetic defect. Statistical analysis supports a recessive inheritance pattern in approximately 10% of men who have aneurysms. Research in this area is active and implicates an autosomal diallelic major locus.

The two genes with the strongest supporting evidence of contribution to the genetic risk for AAA are the CDKN2BAS gene, also known as ANRIL, which encodes an antisense ribonucleic acid that regulates expression of the cyclin-dependent kinase inhibitors CDKN2A and CDKN2B, and DAB2IP, which encodes an inhibitor of cell growth and survival. Functional studies are now needed to establish the mechanisms by which theses genes contribute toward AAA pathogenesis [17].

Structural pathophysiology

Atherosclerosis

The traditional view of aneurysm formation is that arterial dilation is a consequence of degenerative atherosclerotic disease, which results in acquired wall weakness. The experienced vascular surgeon is well aware that peripheral arteriosclerosis and aneurysmal disease often coexist. Severe atherosclerotic calcification in the aortoiliac vessels presents a technical challenge in aneurysm surgery. Epidemiologic, radiographic, and histologic data support the association between aneurysm disease and atherosclerosis [18].

AAAs and atherosclerosis share many risk factors and frequently occur simultaneously. The frequency of aortic aneurysms closely parallels the prevalence of atherosclerosis; for example, the low abdominal aneurysm rate in Asia correlates with the decreased incidence of atherosclerosis. Radiographic and histopathologic studies support the link between atherosclerosis and aneurysms. Ultrasound screening of patients with peripheral vascular disease detects a 5.9% rate of AAA, double that of the general population [19]. Studies of patients suffering from coronary and carotid artery occlusive disease detect an aortic aneurysmal rate of 11–13.5% [9]. Histologic evaluations of sections from aortic aneurysms show atherosclerotic changes and thinning of the media.

Pathophysiologic principles also support the concept that atherosclerosis contributes to aneurysm formation. Atherosclerotic plaques may obstruct nutrient diffusion from the lumen to the media. The needs of the media must then be supplied exclusively by vasa vasorum from the adventitia. However, this may be inadequate due to incomplete distribution of vasa vasorum throughout the human arterial system [20]. Aortic vasa vasorum usually arise from the renal arteries, accounting for the relative sparing of the perirenal aorta from aneurysm formation.

Structural changes induced by atherosclerosis may contribute to aneurysm formation. As atherosclerosis progresses in humans, friable type I collagen replaces native type III collagen [21].Thus, the architectural integrity of the vessel is impaired, leading to a predilection to aneurysm formation. An association between aortic aneurysms and atherosclerosis is not surprising since the geometry and hemodynamics of arterial dilation predispose to atherosclerosis formation. Aneurysms have increased in incidence, prevalence, and mortality over the last 30 years, while coronary artery and cerebrovascular diseases have not. The divergence of these diseases in prevalence and mortality indicates that while risk factors are shared, the development of aneurysm disease is not entirely explained by atherosclerosis.

Although the epidemiologic link between the two is strong, it is propose that occlusive atherosclerotic aortic disease and aortic aneurysmal disease are distinct entities [12]. This is based on the different characteristics of these groups including age of onset, male–female ratio, clinical course, and prognosis. Evidence found to correlate with the size and state of aneurysm indicates that aneurysms reflect a heterogeneous disease with multiple forms and etiologic factors.

Autoimmunity

Autoimmunity may precipitate the inflammatory cascade. Aneurysm aortic extract was studied and noted to contain large quantities of IgG. Further studies revealed that the IgG from AAA patients was present and reactive against various proteins present in the aneurysmal aorta [22]. One of the initial putative autoantigen extracts was an 80-kDa dimer, designated aortic aneurysm associated protein-40 (AAAP-40). AAAP-40 was reactive with 79% (11 of 14) of AAA IgG preparations, and 11% (1 of 9) of controls (p = 0.002) (Gregory). Other autoantigens have subsequently been found, and are currently under investigation in our laboratory. Evidence continues to accumulate to support the notion that autoimmunity may play an important role in aneurysmal degeneration of the aorta. Some of these autoantigens are absent in the external iliac artery, perhaps explaining why this artery rarely becomes aneurismal.

Triggering of autoimmunity can be brought about by autoantigens or molecular mimics. For example, molecular mimicry may occur with cytomegalovirus and clone 1. Also, rabbit antibody against Treponemapallidumand herpes simplex have been shown to bind to the adventitial elastin-associated microfibrils. The putative autoantigen AAAP-40 has homologies with Treponemapallidumand herpes. The hypothesis is that there are epitopes in the microbial proteins that are similar to the AAAP-40, thereby triggering an autoimmune response. Tanaka et al [23] detected herpes simplex viral DNA in 12 of 44 AAA specimens, compared with 1 of 10 normal subjects.

Inflammation

The normal aorta has few inflammatory cells within in its wall. An influx of CD3+ cells and lymphocytes is seen in AAA tissues Although 66% of all lymphocytes in AAAs are in the adventitia, polyclonal B-lymphocytes are abundant in the media. IgG is elevated in AAA specimens. In [24] it was showed an inflammatory infiltrate in the adventitia in 68% of 156 AAA resection specimens examined retrospectively. Macrophages are found throughout the wall of AAA specimens. The macrophage Fc receptors regulate the secretion of proteinases by receptor specific mechanisms. Phagocytes produce proteinases such as elastase and collagenase. On the other hand, it have been implicated the collagenase, stromelysin, and gelatinase-B (MMP-1,3,9) in the destruction of the aorta matrix [25]. Cytokines are released by inflammatory cells and smooth muscle cells in the aorta. They are predominantly: interleukin 1 (IL-1), IL-6, IL-8, monocyte chemoattractant protein (MCP-1), tumor necrosis factor (TNF), and interferon (IFN). These cytokines, to varying degrees, cause MMP expression, TIMP reduction, induction of prostaglandin synthesis, lymphocyte proliferation, and chemotaxis. An autoimmune or inflammatory cascade, as proposed in some etiologies of AAAs, is perpetuated via the use of cytokines [26].

Enzymatic degradation

The elastin: collagen ratio has consistently been shown to be reduced in AAAs when ompared with normal aortas, leading to loss of elasticity and weakening of the aneurysmal wall. This may not be simply due to increased elastin degradation, as Minion et al. have shown that the total elastin content of the aneurismal wall may actually increase, but that the corresponding increase in collagen is much greater (Minion). Despite this evidence, there is little doubt that proteolysis plays an important role in aneurysm development. Aneurysmal disease differs from stenotic disease by the intensity of proteolytic activity within the extracellular matrix. The established association with chronic lung disease supports the argument that elastolysis is a major contributory factor, and indeed this is an area in which there has been much research. For some time, the cause of elastin degradation remained unknown, but even as early as 1980 when it was described increased collagenase activity [27]. In 1991, it was found a spectrum of collagenase activity in the aortic wall of both atherosclerotic and aneurysmal vessels ranging from 55–92 kDa [29].

Importantly, although the collagenase activity was limited, it increased dramatically when tissue inhibitors of metalloproteinases (TIMPs) were destroyed. In [30], it wasalso described the increased expression of a 92 kDagelatinase in AAAs when compared with both normal aortas and aorto-occlusive disease, and localized this to the area around infiltrating macrophages. This gelatinase is part of a family of zinc-dependent proteolytic enzymes, the matrix metalloproteinases (MMPs), now known as MMP9. In the same year, Freestone et al [31],further elucidated the relative amounts of both MMP9 and MMP2 by a combination of gelatinzymography and immunoblotting. This study demonstrated that the principal gelatinase in smaller aneurysms was MMP2, but that in larger aneurysms MMP9 predominated. McMillan et al [21],investigated mRNA levels for MMPs in AAAs and found that MMP9 was maximally expressed in moderate diameter (5–6.9 cm) rather than large (>7 cm) or small (<4 cm) aneurysms. These findings suggested that whilst MMP9 was responsible for the rapid growth that was seen in this size of aneurysm, other enzymes were responsible for initiation and rupture. Pyoet al.'s paper elegantly proves a link between MMP9 and aneurysm pathogenesis by looking at the effect of inhibiting it both pharmacologically and by targeted gene disruption [32]. Mice that were deficient in the MMP9 gene failed to develop aneurysms as their wild-type counterparts did when subjected to elastase perfusion of the aorta. Bone marrow transplants from each group to the other reversed the response to elastase infusion, demonstrating that the expression of MMP9 by inflammatory cells is crucial to aneurysm development. Other MMPs have also been implicated in the development of AAAs, particularly MMP1 and MMP3. Vine and Powell also found immunoreactive MMP1 in extracts from AAAs (Vine). And more recently the expression of MMP3, as measured by reverse transcriptase polymerase chain reaction (rt-PCR), was found to be elevated in AAAs when compared to aorto-occlusive disease.

Matrix metalloproteinase 13 is a recently described enzyme also known as collagenase-3 and its expression is tightly regulated. Whilst MMP13 was not expressed at all in normal tissue, it was found in atherosclerotic disease and in significantly higher concentrations in AAAs. Expression was localized to medial smooth muscle cells in the aortic tissue, and could also be detected in human vascular smooth muscle cells in culture. Membrane type MMP1 (MT MMP1) is an activator of MMP2 and was found to be increased in aneurismal aorta when compared to normal or atherosclerotic aorta. Membrane type MMP1 was localized to aortic smooth muscle cells and macrophages in aneurysmal tissue by immunohistochemical analysis. The ability to activate MMP2 was confirmed by the addition of radiolabelled pro-MMP2, and determination of the subsequent amount of radiolabelled active MMP2. In vivo, the activity of MMPs is tightly controlled by their natural inhibitors, the TIMPs. In 2000, it was demonstrated that TIMP-1 bound to both the monomeric and dimeric forms of MMP9, whereas TIMP-2 bound only to the active form. Whilst it has been shown that the TIMPs are present in large quantities in AAAs, it has been suggested that itis an imbalance between MMPs and TIMPs that leads to the net increase in proteolysis seen. Tamarinaet al also showed that the TIMP: MMP ratio was actually decreased in AAAs, despite an absolute increase in TIMP levels [33].

Whilst there has been considerable work published in the area of collagenases and other metalloproteinases in AAAs, less is known about the role of serine proteases. Elastases of approximately 20–30 kDa have been demonstrated in the inner aspect of the media in AAAs. This elastase works best in the alkaline range, and is inhibited by α-1 anti-trypsin. The fact that it is also inhibited by phenylmethylsulphonyl fluoride (PMSF) confirms that it is indeed a serine protease. Five distinct serine proteases have been separated by gel electrophoresis from aortic aneurysm tissue, suggesting there is a spectrum of enzymes at work. In addition to MMPs and serine proteases, there is also the cysteine protease group. These differ from serine proteases by the substitution of an Asn residue for an Asp in the catalytic triad. Cathepsins S and K are examples of this type of elastase and have been shown to be produced in abundance by smooth muscle cells in atheroma. They are inhibited by cystatin C, the expression of which is governed by a polymorphism of its signal peptide. As discussed previously, patients in whom the cathepsins were not inhibited displayed faster growing aneurysms.

AAA is a multifactorial disease with genetic risk factors and an immunologic component. Immune cells, including macrophages, neutrophils, mast cells, B- and T- lymphocytes, along with vascular smooth muscle cells and adventitial fibroblasts, produce cytokines and enzymes, promoting an inflammatory reaction, extracellular matrix degradation, and neovascularization. Among the different enzymes secreted by immune and stromal cells, matrix metalloproteinase (MMP)-2, MMP-9, MMP-12, cathepsins, and neutrophil elastase cause medial degeneration. Chymase causes smooth muscle cell apoptosis, and MMP-3, MMP-8, and MMP-13 cause adventitial collagen degradation, promoting abdominal aortic aneurysm rupture [34].

Oxidative stress

The action of reactive oxygen species has been implicated in the etiology of many disease processes. In particular, the effect of oxidative stress on many aspects of vascular biology has come under intense scrutiny over the past few years. The addition of antioxidants significantly reduced the activity of MMP9, whereas the addition of inhibitors of protein kinase C had no effect. These results suggest that the increased proteolytic activity seen in the extracellular matrix in patients with diabetes mellitus is due, at least in part, to the effects of oxidation, and may help to explain a link between aneurysm formation and oxidative stress. A further series of aortic banding experiments have demonstrated that in areas of high pressure there is an up-regulation of endothelial nitric oxide synthase (eNOS) when compared with tissues downstream of the artificial coarctation [35].

Measuring nitrotyrosine in the same tissues gave some indication of the degree of nitric oxide breakdown and sequestration by reactive oxygen species. In the areas above the banding (heart, brain and thoracic aorta) the levels of nitrotyrosine were much higher than in areas not exposed to high pressures (distal aorta). The inactivation of nitric oxide due to oxidative damage in areas of high pressure is another indication of vascular endothelial dysfunction, which may contribute to the pathogenesis of aneurysms. Combining the in vitro elastase perfusion rat model of Anidjaret al [10],with modern cDNAmicroassay analysis,looked at the expression of 8799 genes in rats with induced aortic aneurysms, and compared them with genes expressed in rats that had undergone sham operations [36]. Using this technique they were able to identify over 200 genes whose expression had more than doubled in the aneurysm group. Significantly, this included many genes reflecting an increase in oxidative stress, notably hemeoxygenase, inducible nitric oxide synthase (iNOS), 12-lipoxygenase and heart cytochrome C oxidase, subunit VIa. Conversely, antioxidant genes such as superoxide dismutase, reduced NAD-cytochrome b-5 reductase and glutathione S reductase werefound to be down-regulated. These two complementary findings both point to oxidative stress playing a major role in AAA development.

Infection

Infected aortic aneurysms are uncommon, and infrequently have their pathological features been described. Panneton and Edwards evaluated clinical and histopathologic features in patients undergoing surgical repair of infected aneurysms of the descending thoracic or abdominal aorta over a 24-year period [37]. The results showed that among cases with an identifiable causative organism, staphylococcus accounted for 30%, streptococcus for 20%, salmonella for 20%, Escherichia coli for 15%, and other organisms for 15%.

During recent years, attention has been paid to the role of atypical bacterial infections, including Chlamydia and Helicobacter pylori, in the process of atherogenesis and arterial disease development. The reported rates of detection within atherosclerotic lesions by PCR vary widely. Regarding Chlamydia, several studies hypothesized this organism as a possible source of vascular disease, including carotid, coronary, and aortic pathology. Its role in the pathogenesis of aortic aneurysms, however, has been controversial. Sodecket al [38],investigated the presence of C. pneumoniae in 148 tissue samples excised from control and diseased aortas. DNA of C. pneumoniae, C. trachomatis and C. psittaci were assessed by highly sensitive and specific real time polymerase chain reaction (PCR). C. trachomatis-DNA was detected in 1/65 diseased patients and in none of 83 controls (P=0.43). In a similar study, surgical specimens derived from aneurysm or aorta fragments were investigated for C. pneumoniae utilizing PCR. In asymptomatic aneurysms, DNA was found in 9 cases (29%), and in ruptured aneurysms in 14 cases (49%). In the control group, C. pneumoniae DNA was not detected in the aortic wall. Conflicting data has failed to show a clear relationship between chlamydia infection and aortic pathology.

Cytomegalovirus (CMV)-induced arterial disease has also been linked to aortic pathology. To further elucidate the mechanism by which CMV may promote atherosclerosis, Westphalet al.(Westhpal), studied the expression pattern of cellular inflammatory and proliferative signals in the aortic wall of CMV (+) and CMV (−) patients undergoing coronary artery bypass grafting (CABG). CMV-DNA in smooth muscle cells was thought to induce local growth factor expression as well as endothelial activation, both of which can promote the progression of atherosclerosis. Since traditional atherogenic risk factors increase the likelihood of aortic CMV manifestation, CMV may play a crucial role in mediating the progression of atherosclerosis. The persistent expression of CMV-gene in the vessel wall plays a role in the vascular cellular response, including progression of atherosclerosis or vasculitis in vivo. Kilicet al [39], performed PCR analysis to demonstrate the relationship between CMV and atheromathosis at the aortic wall. CMV DNA was found in 37.9% atherosclerotic and 32.7% non-atherosclerotic vascular wall specimens.

Vitamin E deficiency

Studies have pointed to an inverse relationship between vitamin E (a-tocopherol) levels and the incidence of arterial disease. Vitamin E is an important lipid-soluble antioxidant that localizes to the hydrophobic area of biologic membranes [40]. In terms of AAA, it is hypothesized that activated polymorphonuclear cells (PMNs) release proteinases which degrade the aortic wall matrix. These same PMNs would also release oxidative enzymes, generating toxic oxygen species such as hydrogen peroxide which would lead to lipid peroxidation. Vitamin E is considered a specific, though indirect, index of in vivo peroxidation. They also showed that a small group of AAA patients had decreased vitamin E levels but not decreased vitamin E/total lipid ratios compared with controls (coronary artery disease and normal patients). Accordingly, the AAA patients may be under increased oxidative stress (e.g., increased inflammation or PMN activation) but do not have decreased concentrations of plasma vitamin E carriers.

This analysis reveals how the biological information associated with AAA pathogenesis constitute the foundation on which can be defined the destructive remodeling of the aortic wall and its influence in AAA rupture.

4. Morphological Biodeterminants, MBDs

After its formation, the aneurysm trends to increase in size and change its shape as consequence of the arterial wall destructive remodeling. This phenomenon, which occurs along many years in asymptomatic way, characterizes the AAA morphology and morphometry. Aneurysm geometric characteristics have been reported to be a significant predictors of the tendency for expansion or subsequent risk of rupture [41, 42] and can be the deciding factors in the clinical management of the disease. The correlation of the rupture risk with the aneurysm geometry has been clearly depicted in cases of intracranial aneurysms, where various shape indices were proven to discriminate sufficiently between rupture and unrupture aneurysms.

For AAAs, a pioneer work to assess the rupture risk based using the biomechanical concept was recently presented [43]. The authors combined geometrical and structural factors to obtain a dimensionless severity parameter, from which, they could estimate the potential risk of a specific aneurysm in any stage of development. Later, this concept it was modified for only considering the main geometric parameters of the aneurysm which can be easily determined by computed axial tomography (CT) or magnetic resonance imaging (MRI) obtained during periodic check-up [44]. The basic idea of the method was to correlate the main simple geometric parameters of the aneurysm in order to obtain the morphologic biomechanical determinants, MBDs. This idea is supported by the hypothesis that the aneurysm shape is strongly related with its rupture potential. Here, it is important to take into consideration that this method is a baseline for the determination of a rupture risk predictor and that such a treatment decision must be made within a reasonable turnaround time. Therefore, the precision of the method should be smaller than the clinical scale of evolution of the pathology and justifies the utilization of the aneurysm morphology based on simple geometric parameters as a rupture risk predictor.

Figure 1 shows an AAA schematic representation where the simple geometric parameters involved in this method are defined. D is the diameter at the plane of maximum diameter, D_L is the lumen diameter, L is the aneurysm length which is measured from proximal neck to distal neck, L_A is the anterior length measured from point of intersection O to anterior wall and L_P is the posterior length measured from point of intersection O to posterior wall. During the follow up treatment the current clinical practice establishes that only three parameters are controlled: sagittal and coronal maximum diameter and length.

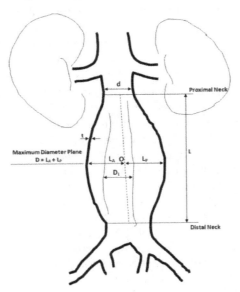

Figure 1. AAA schematic representation with the main geometric parameters.

After careful analysis, these simple parameters have adequately been combined to define the proposed geometric biomechanical factors. Some considerations about them are listed below:

1.   Deformation Rate, χ.Characterizes the actual deformation of the aorta. It is defined as a ratio between the maximum transverse diameter D and infra-renal aorta diameter, d.

This concept considers that the aorta diameters range between 1.5 and 2.5 cm for any patient. The value that defines a low rupture risk is taken as the lower deformation condition of the artery (lower values D and higher d), and for the most critical condition, as the higher deformation (higher values D and lower d).

2.   Asymmetry, β.A characteristic feature of an aneurysm is its asymmetry, which can be attributed to the non-symmetry expansion of the aneurysm sac as a result of the expansionconstraints introduced by the proximity to the spinal column. Due to this, AAA geometry exhibits a high surface complexity and a significant tortuosity of the inflow conduit and the segments of the iliac arteries. An aneurysm has lower rupture risk if it is more symmetric (β=1) and the risk increases as L_P tends to be lower than L_A, which means that β trend to 0.

3.   Saccular Index, γ. This factor assesses the portion of the aorta, with length (L), which is affected by the formation and further development of the aneurysm. This means that long aneurysms have more rupture possibilities than a short one. Typical values of L are ranged from 90 to 140 mm (some works have reported values of L, higher). The calculation condition of the upper threshold value is the higher value of L and the peak value of D (typical for elective repair).

4.   Relative Thickness, ι. The aneurysm geometric characterization determines the existence of a variable wall thickness; both between the anterior and posterior walls and between the aneurysmatic sac and the regions close to the distal and proximal ends.⊙ Initial studies have used uniform wall thickness in their attempt to characterize aneurysm shape. Although wall thickness was not one of the highest ranked features chosen with the feature selection algorithm based on the χ^2–test, its effect on aneurysm rupture cannot be ignore [45]. Typical values of wall thickness (t) in aneurysmatic arteries are ranged from 0.5 to 1.5 mm [46]. This general range may vary from 0.23 mm to 4.26 mm at a calcified site [47]. The danger of aneurysm rupture will be greater when the thickness is low in the peak diameter region. This trend falls with the increase of the wall thickness.

5.   ILT/AAA area ratio,λ. Although 70% of AAA includes thrombus [48], there isnot consensus about its real influence in the AAA rupture phenomenon. Some investigators state that ILT may reduce the stress in the AAA wall, improving its compliance and significantly preventing AAA rupture. Other declared that ILT could accelerate AAA rupture. Hence, it is very important to consider the effects of ILT in the rupture potential, by means of the parameter ILT/AAA area ratio.

6.   Growth rate,ε.It is considered as an important indicator for AAA rupture. A high expansion rate of 0.5-1.0 cm/year is often associated with a high risk of rupture, and an elective repair should be considered even if the maximum diameter is lower than 5 cm. The value indicating that an aneurysm is in rupture risk has been determined regarding to the worst situation (the lowest value inside the range of high growth rate (0.5cm/year), the peak diameter D and the time T between periodic check-up (0.5 year). The low rupture risk limits were determined for aneurysm formation conditions.

Once these factors were defined, it was necessary to evaluate their weight in the rupture phenomenon by means of the definition of the weighted coefficient ωi and of the weighted level risk WLRi.

The weighted coefficient takes into consideration the weight of a specific factor on the frequency of occurrence of the AAA rupture. The initial values of the coefficients ωi have been obtained from the opinion of a group of surgeons about the importance of each factor. Furthermore, the weighted level risk considers the impact of a factor in the probability of AAA rupture and was sorted in four intervals: low impact, middle, high and dangerous. The WLRi have been obtained from considerations made in open literature when the importance of a factor's value is given according to the level of risk.

Table 1 shows the threshold values assigned to each geometric biomechanical factor and their related weighted coefficient and level risk.

| MDDs | Definition | Threshold values | | | | Weighted Coefficient, ωi |
		Low Risk	Middle Risk	High Risk	Dangerous	
Deformation Rate, χ	$\dfrac{D}{d}$	1.20-1.70	1.71-2.30	2.31-3.29	≥ 3.3	0.35
Asymmetry, β	$\dfrac{(D - L_A)}{L_A}$	1-0.9	0.8-0.7	0.6-0.5	≤ 0.4	0.10
Saccular Index, γ	$\dfrac{D}{L}$	≥ 0.75	0.74-0.69	0.68-0.61	≤ 0.6	0.10
ILT/AAA ratio, λ	$\dfrac{(D^2 - D_L^2)}{D^2}$	0.1-0.24	0.25-0.44	0.45-0.61	≥ 0.62	0.10
Relative Thickness, ι	$\dfrac{t}{D}$	0.05-0.04	0.04-0.02	0.02-0.11	≤ 0.01	0.10
Growth rate, ε	$\dfrac{(D_A - D_P)}{T}$	0.1-0.17	0.18-0.3	0.31-0.49	≥ 0.5	0.25
Weighted Level Risk, WLRi		0.1	0.3	0.7	1	

Table 1. Geometric biomechanical factors characterization.

Hence, rupture risk quantitative indicator defined in term of AAA morphology, can be expressed as the sum of each weighted coefficient ωi multiplied by the corresponding WLRi:

$$RI(t) = \sum_1^6 \omega_i WLR_1 \qquad (1)$$

Regarding the results of RI(t), it is possible to advise several actions and suggestions to physicians. This is shown in Table 2.

As above indicated, the proposed method is based on six geometric biomechanical factors. But, it is possible that, for any reason, the information about some parameters is not available. In this case, the method fits its algorithm to calculate only the factors associated with the existing geometric parameters and it is able to weights the final result according to the amount of parameters taken into account.

An initial limitation of the method is associated with indirect errors in obtaining the MBDs, due to the difficulty in extracting exact values from the geometric parameters needed in determining these MBDs. The measurements of the simple geometric parameters is, usually, carried out by a radiologist, a human being with its professional customs and resources,

RI(t)	Actions/Suggestions
< 0.2	Rupture risk is very low. No action is suggested.
0.2 ÷ 0.45	Rupture risk is low. A close observation is required.
÷ 0.7	Elective repair should be considered. Other symptoms such a back and abdominal pain, syncope or vomiting, should be observed.
> 0.7	Rupture risk is very high. Surgical intervention must be necessary.

Table 2. RI(t) intervals and actions and suggestions offered by method to physicians.

with best and/or worst days, with/without personal and labor problems. Therefore, it is important to assess the influence of all these (and others) conditions on the precision of the results.

The ANSI-ASME PTC 85, ISSO 5167 standard was used to determine the indirect errors in the calculation of GBDs due to the direct measurements of the simple geometric parameters. The methodology was applied to data-base which was used for validation tests. The results that are shown in Table 3 correspond to higher values for the errors obtained. The bias limit in measuring of the geometric parameters for all parameters was considered 0.001m. The main conclusion that can be drawn from Table 3 is that the errors in determining the MBDs, are not significant.

MDBs	Uncertainty, Uz	Relative uncertainty, U (%)
Deformation Rate, χ	1.81E-01	0.0464
Asymmetry, β	2.55E-02	0.075
Saccular Index, γ	1.23E-02	0.022
ILT/AAA ratio, λ	1.81E-03	3.13E-03
Relative Thickness, ι	1.18E-02	1.8
Growth rate, ε	1.67E-02	0.027

Table 3. Indirect errors obtained in determining the GBDs.This standard allows defining the experimental uncertainty, U in determining a variable Z, as:

This initial set of values was validated by using one clinical case and three cases from literature.

In shortly. In the clinical case, the state of a 74 year-old male patient with an aneurysm was assessed. The geometrical characterization shows that the peak diameter is lower than the threshold value (50 mm), therefore under current medical practice; the patient should be kept under observation. But, on the other hand, the values of the deformation rate and the asymmetry index fall into the high risk level interval. It must be noticed that by means of statistical analysis these geometric biomechanical factors are considered as the most influential factors on the aneurysm potential rupture.Other two MBDs are also sorted as high risk level, although their weight on the rupture phenomenon is lower. Therefore, the value of the patient-specific quantitative predictor calculated by equation (1) is RI(t)=0.64, which indicates that the elective repair should be considered. This result was confirmed because, during the period of check-up examination, the patient underwent an emergency surgical procedure for aneurysm rupture in the posterior wall.

In another test, a triple validation was performed comparing the results documented in the original papers [49], [50] and [51], the results presented by [43] and the results obtained with the proposed set of values [52]. The geometries of the different analyzed AAAs are very different, however the value of RI(t) is able to sort patients correctly. In the model presented in [49], it is noticed that the aneurysm affects a significant region of the aorta and has a high rate of growth, which has a high relative importance in the value of $RI(t)$. In the model [50], the two biomechanical factors that have more influence in the deterioration of the aneurysm increase in comparison with the previous one, but they stay in the range of elective repair, although it was expected that the indicator value would be higher.

Analyzing the model [51], it is noticed that there is a worsening of most of the geometric parameters; the most important are a high growth rate, a maximum diameter 20% greater than the threshold value and an aneurysm affecting a significant region of the artery. This behavior justifies that the value of the rupture risk indicator falls into the category of possible rupture.

These results encouraged the implementation of another validation test: a broader control study with a population of two hundred and one patients at the Clinic Hospital of Valladolid-Spain, who were submitted to Endovascular Aneurysm Repair (EVAR) treatment.Previously, a new the set of values for the weighted coefficient was defined by using a statistical tool to contrast the hypothesis that certain events have a probability of occurring. In this case, the event is associated to the AAA rupture due to a specific MBD.

According to this statistical tool, the new set of values resulting for ωi is: Deformation Rate= 0.35, Asymmetry=0.07, Saccular Index=0.1, Relative Thickness=0.07, ILT/AAA area ratio=0.07 and Growth rate=0.34.

For this new test, the population of the sample was divided in three groups: Group I (n=174) - patients without later consequences after EVAR treatment; Group II (n=5) - patients who died from causes associated with the AAA pathology; Group III (n=22) - patients whose AAA ruptures. As all these patients were submitted to EVAR treatment, the main objective of this test is to verify if some of the surgical procedures in patients whose aneurysm has a maximum diameter higher than threshold value could have been avoided, and/or if the method can predict the rupture of aneurysm with a diameter less than the threshold value.

The results showed that in 88% of the patients who belongs to group I is justified the surgical procedure, because the $RI(t)$ values fall into dangerous and high level rupture risk. In the group II, the results suggest that the five patients should be submitted to surgical procedure because their rupture risk index is dangerous + high risk condition. All these patients died either during repair treatment or during recovering of it. The state of health of all these patients was not good, because they presented other diseases like renal chronic insufficiency, atheromatic plaque, previous complications related with cardiovascular diseases, digestive hemorrhages.

Very interesting results are obtained in the analysis of the group III. The values of *RI(t)* indicate that95.4% of the patients, present levels of rupture risk sorted as dangerous and high and the surgical procedure could have been considered before rupture. All these patients had aneurysms whose maximum diameter was less than the threshold value for surgical treatment and a systematic (time between two consecutive revisions lower than 1 year) follow-up check are suggested to diminishing the risks associated to emergency surgery by ruptures.

The fact that one patient presented a middle rupture index was somewhat unexpected and it is probably attributable to a combination of other factors not considered here, associated to factors of biological and/or structural nature. It was verified that the geometric parameters are lower than the threshold values.

The obtained outcomes are promising and have motivated further actions. Recent studies [53] have identified other MBDs based on the lumen centerline geometry. According to [54], the resulting centerline is a piecewise linear line defined on the Voronoi diagram, whose vertices lie on Voronoi polygon boundaries [55]. Values of Voronoi sphere radius $R(x)$ are therefore defined on centerlines, so that centerline points are associated with maximal inscribed spheres. Since centerlines were constructed to lie on local maxima of distance from the boundary, there is a tight connection between maximal sphere radius and minimum projection diameter used in clinical evaluation. In fact, classic angiographic vessel diameter evaluation is performed considering the minimum diameter obtained by measurements on different projections. The availability of a robust method for centerline computation and diameter measurement allows to characterize blood vessel geometry in a synthetic way, therefore giving the opportunity of performing a study on a population of models. Since it has been shown that planarity, tortuosity and branching angles have a major influence on complex blood flow patterns, such a study may reveal if particular vessel configurations are involved in vascular pathology.

Three MBDs have been defined using this approach: tortuosity, curvature and torsion centerline. Today, VMTK software havebeen developed to 3D reconstruction of the lumen centerline geometry. Figure 2 shows the visual representation of these determinants. Tortuosity, an absolute number, expresses the fractional increase in length of a tortuous vessel in relation to the imaginary straight line and has been described in [55]. Torsion is measured in $1/cm^2$ and curvature is measured in $1/cm$.

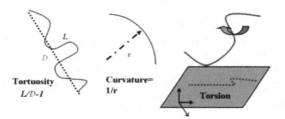

Figure 2. Schematic visualization of tortuosity, curvature and torsion [53].

Recently, it has been postulated that aneurysm peak wall stress (PWS) may be superior to diameter as predictor of the rupture risk. This statement has its theoretical foundation in the physical principle of the aneurysm rupture. Complex AAA geometry contributes to equivalent complex wall stress distribution over the entire AAA, with the higher stresses associated with regions of high curvature [56].

The role of these geometric biodeterminants in the prediction of AAA it has been assessed taking into consideration the presence of intra-luminal thrombus (ILT) [53]. In the study were included nineteen patients whose-which AAA maximum diameters ranged from 5 to 12 cm. Statistical analysis confirmed that the maximum diameter significantly influenced PWS and the tortuosity may also affect PWS values in models with ILT in the same direction.

On the other hand, it has been demonstrated [57] that PWS is strongly correlated with the maximum diameter as well as the centreline asymmetry. It is notable, however, that in 73% of the analyzed models in this work a significant correlation was found between asymmetry and maximum diameter. Therefore, if diameter strongly correlated with peak stress then asymmetry would also score high.

Perhaps one of the most ambiguous issues in the assessment of rupture risk is the existence as well as the develop of the ILT. Despite ILT's impact on aneurysm disease, little is known about its development, and it is unclear whether it increases or decreases the risk of aneurysm rupture. That is, the ILT reinforces proteolytic activity [58], which weakens the wall [59], or buffers against wall stress [50]. It has been hypothesized that ILT develops either from rupture of vulnerable plaques or as a more continuous process characterized by blood-flow induced activation of platelets and their deposition at non-endothelialized sites of the wall exposed to low (sub-physiological) wall shear stress [60].

Recently, the investigationsare addressed to the integration of ILT in the computational models and, consequently, its effects in patient-specific on PWS values and distribution. A significant difference in PWS when including the ILT in 3D AAA computational model it has been reported [61]. Wang et al [50] showed that computational integration of ILT in 3D models could actually modify not only the value but also the distribution of PWS, thus playing a protective role against rupture but this conclusion was not supported in [62]. On the other hand, there is still some concern regarding the protective role of ILT, since many authors who evaluate the influence of ILT on hemodynamic stress transmission, reported that he presence of ILT fails to reduce the transmission of this stress on the AAA wall, consequently, leaving the AAA rupture risk equalled [63]. AAAs can experience higher stresses at regions of inflection, regardless of wall thickness variation. In such cases, the concentric or eccentric location of ILT in the AAA sac cannot be effectively reduce PWS values or changes its distribution [64]. A question of interest arises here, regarding whether such PWS values derived from computational estimation should be taken into consideration, since AAA rupture rarely takes places at these sites, reserving this possibility only for thrombosed AAAs [65]. Therefore, all these ideas reinforce the need to quantify and take into consideration the effect of the ILT.

Finally, it is important to address the topic related to the use either simple geometric parameters or biodeterminants in the AAA rupture risk assessment. To answer this question some aspects should be analyzed. The first one is related to the temporal scales of the disease progression which is higher than the results' precision in the determination of the geometric parameters. This conclusion justify the use of morphological determinants. On the other hand, is the fact that aneurysm shape has a significant influence on flow patterns and consequently in its rupture potential. Recent findings have shown that the aneurysm geometrical shape may be related to the rupture risk. The morphological nature determinants (MBDs) are defined by appropriate relations among simple geometric parameters to characterize the influence of the aneurysm morphology on its rupture potential.

Utilizing idealized aneurysm models of the true vessel lumen surface geometry, the role of the geometric characteristics in the hemodynamic stresses prediction by using of Pearson's rank correlation coefficients was assessed [66]. In this work, the model was modified to allow the parametrization of the main parameters assessed: maximum diameter D, length L and asymmetry, β. Figure 3, shows a schematic view of the models used in this study.

The results show that hemodynamics stresses correlate better with MBDs. For hemodynamic pressure, the relation with saccular index and deformation rate are strong and negative (r=-0.75, p=0.000 and r=-0.7, p=0.000 respectively). The asymmetry coefficient has no-significant correlation (r=-0.25, p=0.00).

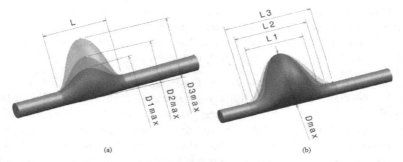

Figure 3. Schematic view of the parametrized aneurysm models. a) L and β are constant and D varies; b) D and β are constant and L varies.

The relation of asymmetry and deformation rate with WSS is weak with significance less than 15% and saccular index is no significant.

The main conclusions of this study are: luminal pressure is the primary mechanical load on the aneurismal wall and that MBDs are better predictors than simple parameters of the hemodynamic stresses.

On the other hand, Raghavanet al [67], showed that the deviation of the aneurysm shape from spherical configuration, the level of its surface ondulation or ellipticity and the norm of the surface mean curvature are a good predictors of rupture.

This analysis confirms that MBDs may become a useful addition to current clinical criteria, mainly maximum diameter, in the decision-making process of the aneurysm treatment. Certainly, as in the same way that other biomechanical consideration, the suggested models require further studies.

5. Structural Biodeterminants, SBDs

In addition to morphological factors, numerically predicted wall stress, finite element analysis rupture index, rupture potential index and severity parameters have been proposed as alternative approaches to assessing rupture risk [68].

The criterion currently used by the medical community is that you can relate directly the risk of rupture with the maximum diameter of the aneurysm. However, as noted above, the biomechanics states that rupture occurs when wall stress exceeds its strength. This assumes a linear relationship between the maximum stress and the maximum diameter of the aneurysm. Thus, we propose an equation to describe this approach.

$$\sigma_{max} = kR_{max} \tag{2}$$

where σ_{max} is the maximum stress in the aneurysm, k is a constant determined by experience, and R_{max} the maximum radius of the aneurysm. The maximum diameter criterion has many limitations.

Since there is currently no method to determine the stresses in the wall in vivo, it is necessary to develop models of the mechanical behavior of the arterial wall. These models can be generated from ideal parameterized geometries created by three-dimensional design software (CATIA, SolidWorks, etc.), or can be obtained through the processing of medical images.

Once the geometry is generated, we calculate using finite element method software (ANSYS, ABAQUS, etc.) in order to determine the stress distribution in the wall of AAA.

Structural biomechanical determinant of VandeGeest

After evaluating the stresses, and using the ultimate strength of arterial tissue or an assessment of the strength of the wall, you can define a structural biomechanical factor. This factor or biodeterminant, can allow us to estimate how close an aneurysm can be of the rupture and, consequently, the appropriateness of the surgical procedure in the patient.

Thus, it is proposed [69] the following factor:

$$RI(t) = \frac{Stress_i}{Strength_i} \tag{3}$$

where i is the chosen point on aneurysm geometry.

It is noted that when the rupture index approaches the value of 1, the state of risk of aneurysm rupture increases, ie when the stress observed in the wall reaches the value of strength.

If the strength is only an estimated value for the entire aneurysm, use the maximum stress given by the simulation. But, when using the strength distribution in the whole geometry, the rupture index is evaluated at each point of the geometry of the aneurysm.

Rupture criterion of Li and Kleinstreuer

This approach [70] is based not only on statistical analysis of some cases of abdominal aortic aneurysms, but also on results of numerical simulations. To do so, tests were conducted with 10 patients whose data were known, in order to verify the accuracy criterion used to calculate σ_{max}:

$$\sigma_{max} = 0.006 \frac{(1-0.68\lambda)e^{\left(0.0123(0.85P_{sist}+19.5D)\right)}}{t^{0.63}\beta^{0.125}} \tag{4}$$

where σ_{max} is the maximum stress that appears frequently in an area whose diameter is equal to two thirds of the maximum diameter of AAA, λ is the ratio of the areas in the plane of maximum diameter ($\lambda = A_{ILT,max} / A_{AAA,max}$), β is the coefficient of asymmetry, P_{sis} is the systolic blood pressure (mmHg), D is the maximum diameter of AAA (cm) and t is the thickness of the wall in the plane of maximum diameter.

If the thickness of the arterial wall cannot be determined from images taken by the TAC, can be approximated by the following equation:

$$t = 3.9 \left(\frac{D}{2}\right)^{-0.2892} \tag{5}$$

According to the authors, this approach presents a very low error in the determination of the maximum stress compared to other models. Whatever the feature is used to calculate stress, the results are very similar to the stress determined by finite element method software.

Clearly, the geometry should not be too complex, which is a limitation. Furthermore, the location of the maximum stress cannot determine, although the value is known.

This approach appears to be quite accurate results, and its application is very simple. So it could be used to determine the maximum stress of the aneurysm with a very simple approach. However, we emphasize that in no other study has been applied.

Rupture criterion based on remodeling history model

These models allow determining a stress value, which is compared with the strength of the arterial wall to evaluate if the break is close or not.

The value of strength can be obtained:

- Form literature, which are based on uni-axial tests aneurysmal tissue of patients.
- By an empirical approach based on an expression that takes into account the patient's personal information.

Criteria based on two-dimensional modeling

- It is a very simple model in two dimensions of the arterial wall;

- The maximum stress is located at the maximum diameter;
- The aneurysm is cylindrical (or spherical);
- Wall thickness constant E;
- Linear elastic behavior.

From these criteria leads to a simple equation that relates the pressure P, the wall thickness t and the maximum radius R_{max} of the aneurysm:

$$\sigma_{max} = P \frac{R_{max}}{t} \tag{6}$$

This modeling, which leads to the stress calculation, presents the following limitations:

- The geometry is very simple, which influences the results.
- Although you can adjust the value of the pressure acting on the wall, assigning the value at the studied patient's blood pressure, stress is always proportional to the radius of the aneurysm.

This approach is similar to the criterion of maximum diameter used today.

Criteria based on three-dimensional modeling

a.   Modeling of material behavior: linear elasticity.

Many authors have used an elastic model of the arterial wall in their research [71, 72]

Commenting on the approach proposed in [73], the authors have attempted to determine the influence of the diameter and symmetry in the mechanical stress of the arterial wall of abdominal aortic aneurysm using an elastic behavior of the wall.

This approach has the merit of taking into account the behavior of the material used, and the authors are aware of the limits of their model, since the aim of their study was to show the influence of symmetry. However, other studies [74, 75] showed that the hyperelastic behavioral model is more suitable for simulating an aneurysm under pressure due to the large strains that can undergo aneurysmal arterial wall (20-40%).

b.   Modeling of material behavior: hyperelasticity.

Given the fact that the tissue of the aneurysmal arterial wall can be deformed the order of 20-40%, the behavior can no longer be considered as elastic.

Hyperelastic materials are characterized by the existence of an energy function W, which depends on the state of deformation.

Tensions can be calculated with this energy function W, which depends on the material, which can be isotropic or anisotropic, which will influence in W.

b.1) Isotropic hyperelasticity

In 1940, Mooney and Rivlin established a behavioral model for the material like rubber, whose behavior is similar to the tissue of the arterial wall due to the incompressibility of both materials.

Heng et al. [76], used the Mooney-Rivlin equation to establish one of the simplest hyperelastic models. The problem with this model with only two parameters is that is more suited to the study of polymers. This law was made by Mooney to model the behavior of rubbers, and it seems too simple for the study of tissues, whose behavior seems much more complex because its composition is not homogeneous.

You can also use a more complex form of Mooney-Rivlin model. In [77] it is performed a study which uses this model and the results seem that calculate appropriately the real tensions of the arterial wall. This form uses 9 parameters addition to the incompressibility parameter.

In 2000, it is defined a mathematical model using a regression from experimental results [75]. This is part of the theory of finite deformations and is based on the first principle of mechanics of continuous media. The assumptions underlying this model were that the wall is non-linear, homogeneous, incompressible and isotropic.

In 2006, this model is modified using another form of the density function [78]. It is observed that for incompressible materials considered, this equation is the same as proposed in [75].

In 2008, it is proposed a model based on the concept of material failure energy Φ [79]. This energy is the maximum amount of energy that the wall can withstand before breaking, because of the deformations. This value depends on the atomic or microscopic structure of the wall of an AAA.

b.2) Anisotropic hyperelasticity

• single transverse anisotropy.

In 1976, Tong and Fung [80], developed a cross-anisotropic hyperelastic model, which allows a behavioral model of the arterial wall aneurysm.

• Anisotropy with two families of fibers
    • Rodríguez anisotropichyperelasticmodel [81];
    • Holzapfel anisotropic hyperelastic model [82]. Proposed model for biological materials with two families of collagen fibers, as they really are the arterial walls.

The anisotropic hyperelastic behavior models better approximate the actual behavior of the aneurysmal arterial wall, but according to the model used, the results can be very different. One can see that the Rodríguez hyperelastic anisotropic model is closer (at the level of stress distribution) to an isotropic hyperelastic that the Holzapfelhyperelastic anisotropic model, as shown in Figure 4.

c.   Fluid-Structure Interaction

All approaches that have been presented are based on the physical principle of fault material of aortic wall. However, all these approaches use a constant pressure value (often the peak systolic pressure), whereas, in reality, not only the pressure varies, but also the blood moves. In an attempt to make models as realistic as possible, we have developed the modeling fluid-structure interaction (FSI), in which the model considers simultaneously the effect of blood flow on the arterial wall and vice versa.

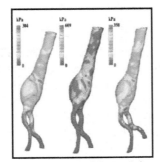

Isotropic Holzapfel Rodríguez

Figure 4. Stress in different models.

Some authors try to use a method of modeling of blood flow, to study its influence on the stresses of the aneurysm wall. These approaches are also used mechanical simulations to assess the stress in the wall of the aneurysm.

From the results obtained with FSI simulations [46], has been determined that in the simulations using the computational analysis of the static stress incurred in an underestimation of wall tension, which is shown in Figure 5. This value can reach 12.5%, as reported [83].

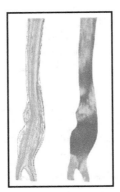

Figure 5. Stream lines which characterize the blood flow inside the aneurysm and surface distribution of stresses, obtained using a modeling FSI.

In 2006, a simulation of aneurysm under pressure [41] and blood flow was carried out in addition to demonstrating that when taking into consideration the bloodstream, the stresses change little while the time required for the simulation is three to four times greater.

The authors concluded that the fluid-structure interaction approach is interesting, but a modeling of the wall with the systolic pressure is sufficient to calculate the stresses in it.

After the revision presented we can conclude that an anisotropic hyperelastic model, using systolic pressure load, and geometry with the important details of the AAA, is the best choice for calculating the stresses in aneurysmal wall.

Evaluation of the arterial wall strength.

At this point, is already known that the evaluation of the wall stress cannot be considered as an isolated indicator to assess the risk of rupture of AAAs, as an aneurysmal wall region which is subjected to high stresses, may also have a high strength, thus equalizing potential rupture. According to the remodeling history model, the strength of the wall is different from patient to patient and in the same patient at different regions and time scales. To resolve this situation, has been developed a technique for noninvasive estimation of the distribution of strength, defining a potential rupture index (RPI)[84], with equation:

$$Strength = 141.26 - 17.16 ILT + 3.39 AGE - 257.3 NORD - 69.5 HIST \qquad (7)$$

where ILT is the thickness of the ILT (in cm), AGE is the patient age in years, $NORD$ is the diameter normalized to the maximum diameter of AAA, $HIST$ is ± ½ according to family history (½ if the history is positive, - ½ if no background) and SEX is ± ½ by sex of the patient (½ if the patient is a man, - ½ for women).

These authors have increasingly improved this criterion, being the last, expressed by equation 8, thatbest approximates the strength of the wall.

$$Strength = 72.9 - 33.5\left((ILT^{0.5}) - 0.79\right) - 12.3(NORD - 2.31) - 24 HIST + 15 SEX \qquad (8)$$

Rupture of aneurysm prediction

The logical process for estimating the risk of aneurysm rupture using structural biomechanical factors would be the one described below:

1. Obtain the blood pressure of the patient.
2. CT of the patient's aneurysm.
3. Geometric model of the aneurysm from medical imaging.
4. Simulation of the aneurysm using data specific to the patient.
5. Estimating the strength of the arterial wall aneurysmal of the patient.
6. State estimation of risk of rupture of the aneurysm.

Subsequently, using the Rupture Index (*RI*) proposed in Equation 1 can be estimated if a ruptured aneurysm is close. Obviously, it will require a medical evaluation of patient state of health (PSH).

Simulation using the Finite Element Method (FEM)

Unable to provide a method for determining the in vivo distribution of wall stress, nowadays it is used the finite element method (FEM), which is recognized as a very precise technique, which aims to find approximate solutions of partial differential equations and integral equations. Equations are solved at the nodes of the meshes that are generated and interpolated within the element, generating a continuous solution throughout the domain.

Overall analysis by using Finite Element Method is an orderly process that will include the following steps:

1. Generation of geometry. The geometry can be generated or imported. In the case of aneurysm geometry is imported directly from the patient CT using some of the commercial software or open source currently available, so it has the actual geometry of the aneurysm affecting the patient under study. Figure 6, shows the geometric model of AAA obtained by the processing of medical images using the public software MeVisLab.

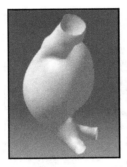

Figure 6. Geometric model of AAA obtained from the processing of medical images.

2. Discretization of meshing domain: The structure or part is divided into elements and modeled as a finite element mesh. In this step the analyst must decide the type, number, size and order of items to be used. This decision will characterize the degree of confidence results thereafter. An example that represents the arterial wall mesh is presented in Figure 7.

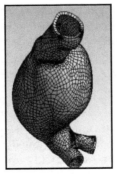

Figure 7. Mesh representation of a geometry that represents the arterial wall of an AAA.

3. Application of the boundary conditions: apply the loads which will be under the model (in this case the blood pressure) and the restrictions of the same (in this case is assumed to be attached to the remainder of the artery limiting their movement and must be taken into account if organs or body parts that limit their movement).

4. Solution of unknown nodal displacements: The global balance equation is modified to take into account the boundary conditions of the problem and to obtain algebraic equations where the unknowns are nodal displacements.
5. Calculation of stresses and strains of the elements: Knowing the nodal displacements resulting from the previous stage, it could be calculated the stresses and strains using the corresponding mechanical equations.
6. Evaluation of results: the stresses solutions are obtained (and displacements in some models) along theaneurysm. It is possible to locate the exact point of the aneurysm where it produces the maximum stress and the value thereof. Figure 8, shows the surface distribution of stresses. The red color indicates the region with higher values of stress and therefore, with greater risk of rupture.

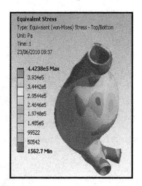

Figure 8. Stress distribution in the arterial wall obtained by finite element simulation.

6. General

At this point, it is important to highlight two aspects. The first one is that the accumulation of knowledge around the topic of accurate prediction of AAA rupture is large enough and significant advances have been achieved in last years although the physicians continue using the same criteria. The second one is related to the growing consensus that it is possible to improve the reliability of the AAA rupture assessment by means of the biomechanical approach.

Despite the growing interest for the behaviour of all these factors, many physicians question its clinical utility advocating the difficulties in its assessing during the everyday clinical practice. Often, these procedures require sophisticated software, very specific and accurate correlations and highly qualified personnel. This feeling appears clearly reflected in a survey carried out among vascular surgeons [85], whose outcomes are summarized in:

90% of the institutions rely their rupture risk estimation on the maximum diameter and the expansion rate, whereas only 15% use the high mechanical stress criteria;

40% of the institutions think that using their criteria, the rupture risk of AAAs is reliable in up to 75% of all cases;

18% of surveyed know and are familiar with the biomechanical criteria to estimate the aneurysm rupture risk, 63% know it but are not familiar with these criteria, where the other percentage has never heard about it.

Seems to be unlikely this knowledge replace the use of current criteria. Clinicians will always feel that large AAAs represent a rupture-threat and should be repaired. It is the small and medium size AAAs that could be examined by using these alternative diagnostic tools which, in the future, may prove to be useful adjunct to maximum diameter.

7. Conclusions

Aneurysmal disease and its progression is a very complex multifactorial process and its statistics are of great concern. The biomechanical approach here developed and substantiated can predict the rupture potential of a patient-specific AAA in any stage of evolution with sufficient accuracy to be clinically relevant. This predictive model is conceived by the integration of biological, morphological and structural information and can constitute a significant step in the clinical management of patients with aneurysm. Nowadays, we are developing a broader validation test of the proposed model by establishing its statistical significance with a large enough number of AAA cases.

Author details

Guillermo Vilalta* and Félix Nieto
Mechanical Engineering Division, CARTIF Centro Tecnológico, Boecillo (Valladolid), Spain

Enrique San Norberto and Carlos Vaquero
Angiology and Vascular Surgery Service,
University and Clinic Hospital of Valladolid, Valladolid, Spain

María Ángeles Pérez
ITAP Institute, University of Valladolid, Valladolid, Spain

José A. Vilalta
Industrial Engineering Department, Polytechnical University of Havana, Havana, 19340, Cuba

8. References

[1] Viceconti M, Taddei F, Van Sint Jan S, Leardini A, Critofolini L, Stea S, Baleani M (2008) MultiscaleModelling of the Skeleton for the Prediction of the Risk of Fracture. Clinical Biomechanics. 23: 845-852.
[2] Newman AB, Arnold AM, Burke GL, O'Leary DH, Manolio TA (2001) Cardiovascular Disease and Mortality in Older Adults with Small Abdominal Aortic Aneurysms Detected by Ultrasonography: the Cardiovascular Health Study. Annals of Internal Medicine. 134: 182–190.

* Corresponding Author

[3] Johansson G, Swedenborg J (1986) Rupture Abdominal Aortic Aneurysms: A Study of Incidence and Mortality. Br. J. Surg. 73: 101-103.

[4] Karkos C, Mukhopadhyay I, Papakostas I, Ghost J, Thomson G, Hughes R (2000) Abdominal Aortic Aneurysm: the Role of Clinical Examination and Opportunistic Detection. Eur. J. Vasc. Endovasc Surg. 19: 299-303.

[5] Vorp DA (2007) Biomechanics of abdominal aortic aneurysm. J. Biomech. 40(9): 1887–1902.

[6] Blanchard JF, Armenian HK, Friesen PP (2000) Risk factors for abdominal aortic aneurysm: results of a case-control study. Am J Epidemiol. 151: 575–83.

[7] Tornwall ME, Virtamo J, Haukka JK, Albanes D, Huttunen JK (2001) Life-style factors and risk for abdominal aortic aneurysm in a cohort of Finnish male smokers. Epidemiology. 12: 94–100.

[8] Singh K, Bonaa KH, Jacobsen BK, Bjork L, Solberg S (2001) Prevalence of and risk factors for abdominal aortic aneurysms in a population-based study: the Tromso study. Am J Epidemiol. 154: 236–244.

[9] Bengtson H, Ekberg O, Aspdlin P, TakoLander R, Bergqvist D (1988) Aneurysmal disease: abdominal aortic dilatation in patients operated on for carotid artery stenosis. Acta Chit Scand. 143: 441-444.

[10] Anidjar S, Osborne-Pellegrin M, Coutard M, Michel JB (1992) Arterial hypertension and aneurismal dilatation. Kidney Int. 37 S61–66.

[11] Johansen K, Koepsell T (1986) Familial tendency for abdominal aortic aneurysms. JAMA. 256: 1934-1936.

[12] Tilson M (1985) Further studies of a putative crosslinking amino acid (3-deoxy-pyridinoline) in skin from patients with AAAs. Surgery. 98: 888-893.

[13] Kitchen ND (1989) Racial distribution of aneurysms in Zimbabwe. JR Soc Med. 82: 136-145.

[14] Webster MW, Ferrel RE, St Jean FL, Majuroder et al (1991) Ultrasound screening of first-degree relatives of patients with abdominal aortic aneurysm. J Vasc Surg. 12: 9-13.

[15] Kuivarilemi H, Tromp G, Prockop DJ (1991) Genetic causes of aortic aneurysms: unlearning at least part of what the textbooks say. J Clin Invest. 88: 1441-1445.

[16] Tromp G, Kuivaniemi H, Shikata H, Prockop DJ (1989) A single basemutation that substitutes serine for glycine 790 of the a 1 (III) chain of type III procollagen exposes an arginine and causes Ehlers–Danlos syndrome IV. J Biol Chem. 264: 1349-1356.

[17] Hinterseher I, Tromp G, Kuivaniemi H (2011) Genes and abdominal aortic aneurysm. Ann Vasc Surg. 25: 388-412.

[18] Nordon IM, Hinghliffe RJ, Holt PJ, et al (2009) Review of current theories for abdominal aortic aneurysm pathogenesis.Vascular. 17: 253-263.

[19] Shapira OM, Pakis S, Wassermann JP, Barzlllai N, Mashlah A (1990) Ultrasound screening for abdominal aortic aneurysms in patients with atherosclerotic peripheral vascular disease. J Cardiovasc Surg. 31: 170-175.

[20] Heistad DD, Marcus ML, Carsen GE et al (1981) Role of vasa vasorum in nourishment of the aortic wall. Am J Physiol. 240: 11781-11783.

[21] McMillan WD, Tamarina NA, Cipollone M (1997) Size matters: the relationship between MMP-9 expression and aortic diameter. Circulation. 96: 2228–2232.

[22] Jagadesham VP, Scott DJ, Carding SR (2008) Abdominal aortic aneurysms: an autoimmune disease? TrensMol Med. 14: 522-529.

[23] Tanaka S, Komori K, et al (1994) Detection of active cytomegalovirus infection n inflammatory aortic aneurysms with RNA polymerase chain reaction. J Vasc Surg. 20: 235-243.

[24] Beckman EN (1986) Plasma cell infiltrates in atherosclerotic in abdominal aortic aneurysms. Am J ClinPathol. 85: 21-24.

[25] Newman KM, Jean-Claude J, et al (1994) Cellular localization of matrix metalloproteinases in the abdominal aortic aneurysm wall. J Vasc Surg. 20: 814-820.

[26] Nanda S, Sharma SG, Longo S (2009) Molecular targets and abdominal aortic aneurysms. Recent Pat Cardiovasc Drug Discov. 4: 150-159.

[27] Busuttil RW, Abou-Zamzam AM, Machleder HI (1980) Collagenase activity of the human aorta. A comparison of patients with and without abdominal aortic aneurysms. Arch Surg. 115: 1373–1378.

[28] Minion DJ, Davis VA, Nejezchleb PA, et al (1994) Elastin is increased in abdominal aortic aneurysms. J Surg Res. 57: 443–446.

[29] Vine N, Powell JT (1991) Metalloproteinases in degenerative aortic disease. Clin Sci. 81: 233–239.

[30] Thompson RW, Holmes DR, Mertens RA et al (1995) Production and localization of 92-kilodalton gelatinase in abdominal aortic aneurysms. An elastolytic metalloproteinase expressed by aneurysm-infiltrating macrophages. J Clin Invest. 96: 318–326.

[31] Freestone T, Turner RJ, Coady A, et al (1995) Inflammation and matrix metalloproteinases in the enlarging abdominal aortic aneurysm. ArterioscThrombVasc Biol. 15: 1145–1151.

[32] Pyo R, Lee JK, Shipley JM, et al (2000) Targeted gene disruption of matrix metalloproteinase-9 (gelatinase B) suppresses development of experimental abdominal aortic aneurysms. J Clin Invest. 105: 1641–1649.

[33] Tamarina NA, McMillan WD, Shively VP, Pearce WH (1997) Expression of matrix metalloproteinases and their inhibitors in aneurysms and normal aorta. Surgery. 122: 264–272.

[34] Rizas KD, ippagunta N, Tilson MD (2009) Immune cells and molecular mediators in the pathogenesis of the abdominal aortic aneurysm. Cardiol Rev. 17: 201-210.

[35] Michel JB, Martin-Ventura JL, Egido J, et al (2011) Novel aspects of the pathogenesis of aneurysms of the abdominal aorta in humans. Cardiovasc Res. 90: 18-27.

[36] Yajima N, Masuda M, Miyazaki M, et al (2002) Oxidative stress is involved in the development of experimental abdominal aortic aneurysm: a study of the transcription profile with complementary DNA microarray. J Vasc Surg. 36: 379–385.

[37] Annambhotla S, Bourgeois S, Wang X, et al (2008) Recent advances in molecular mechanisms of abdominal aortic aneurysm formation. World J Surg. 32: 976-986.

[38] Sodeck G, Domanovits H, Khanakah G, et al (2004) The role of Chlamydia pneumoniae in human aortic disease-a hypothesis revisited. Eur J VascEndovasc Surg. 28: 547–552.

[39] Kilic A, Onguru O, Tugcu H, et AL (2006) Detection of cytomegalovirus and Helicobacter pylori DNA in arterial walls with grade III atherosclerosis by PCR. Pol J Microbiol. 55: 333–337.

[40] Sakalihasan N, Pincemail J, et al (1996)   Decrease of plasma vitamin E (alpha-Tocopherol) levels in patients with abdominal aortic aneurysm. Ann NY Acad Sci. 800: 278-282.

[41] Leung JH, Wright AR, Cheshire N, Crane J, Thom SA, Hughes AD, Xu Y (2006) Fluid structure interaction of patient specific abdominal aortic aneurysms: a comparison with solid stress models. BioMedical Engineering OnLine. http://www.biomedical-engineering-online.com/content/5/1/33. Accessed: 2011 Dec 21.

[42] Vorp DA, VandeGeest JP (2005) Biomechanical determinants of abdominal aortic aneurysm rupture. Arteriosclerosis, Thrombosis, and Vascular Biology. 25: 1558-1566

[43] Kleinstreuer C, Li Z (2006) Analysis and computer program for rupture-risk prediction of abdominal aortic aneurysms. BioMedical Engineering OnLine.Available: http://www.biomedical-engineering-online.com/content/5/1/19. Accessed: 2010 April 15.

[44] Vilalta G, Nieto F, Vaquero C, Vilalta JA (2010) Quantitative Indicator of Abdominal Aortic Aneurysm Rupture Risk Based on its Geometric Parameters, World Academy of Science, Engineering and Technology: 70: 181-185.

[45] Shum J, Martufi G, DiMartino E et al (2011) Quantitative assessment of abdominal aortic aneurysm geometry. [45] Ann. Biomed Eng. 39: 277-286. doi:10.1007/s10439-010-0175-3.

[46] Scotti, CM, Shkolnik AD, Muluk SC, Finol EA (2005) Fluid-structure interaction in abdominal aortic aneurysms: Effects of asymmetry and wall thickness. Biomedical Engineering OnLine.
http://www.biomedical-engineering-online.com/content/4/1/64.Accessed: 2012 Jan 21.

[47] Raghavan ML, Kratzberg J, de Tolosa EMC, et al (2006) Regional distribution of wall thickness and failure properties of human abdominal aortic aneurysm. J. Biomech. 39: 3010-3016.

[48] Frauenfelder T, Boutsianis E, Alkadhi H, Marincek B, Schertler T (2007) Simulation of blood flow within the abdominal aorta. Computational fluid dynamics in abdominal aortic aneurysms before and after interventions.Radiologe. 47: 1021-1028.

[49] M. Raghavan, D. Vorp, M. Federle, M. Makaroun, & M. Webster, Wall stress distribution on three-dimensionally reconstructed models of human abdominal aortic aneurysm. Journal of Vascular Surgery, 31, 2000, 760–769.

[50] D. Wang, M. Makaroun, M. Webster, & D. Vorp, Effect of intraluminal thrombus on wall stress in patient specific model of abdominal aortic aneurysm. Journal of Vascular Surgery, 3, 2002, 598–604.

[51] K. Wilson, A.J. Lee, P.R. Hoskins, F.G. Fowkers, C.V. Ruckley, & A.W. Bradbury, The relationship between aortic wall distensibility and rupture of infrarenal abdominal aortic aneurysm. Journal of Vascular Surgery, 37, 2003, 112–117.

[52] Vilalta G, Nieto F, Vilalta JA et al (2012) Predicción del riesgo de ruptura de aneurismas de aorta abdominal. Método basado en los biodeterminantes geométricos. DYNA Ingeniería e Industria. 87: 66-73. doi: http://dx.doi.org/10.6036/4145.

[53] Georgakaratos E, Ioannou CV, Kamarianakis Y, Papaharilaou Y, Kostas T, Manousaki E, Katsamouris AN (2010) The role of geometric parameters in the prediction of abdominal aortic aneurysm wall stress. Eur. J. VascEndovasc Surg. 39: 42-48.

[54] Antigua L. Patient-Specific Modeling of Geometry and Blood Flow in Large Arteries. Ph.D thesis.Politecnico di Milano 2002

[55] L. Antiga, B. Ene-Iordache, and A. Remuzzi (2003) Computational geometry for patient-specific reconstruction and meshing of blood vessels from MR and CT angiography. IEEE Transactions on Medical Imaging. 22: 674-684.

[56] Thomas JB, Antigua L, Che SL, Milner JS et al. Variation in the carotid bifurcation geometry of younger versus older adults. Stroke, 36: 2450-2456, 2005.

[56] Sacks MS, Vorp ML, RaghavanM;Federle MP, Webster MW (1999) In vivo three-dimensional surface geometry of abdominal aortic aneurysms. Ann. Biomed. Eng. 27:469-479.

[57] Doyle BJ, Eng AC, Burke PE, et al (2009) Vessel asymmetry as an additional diagnostic tool in the assessment of abdominal aortic aneurysm. J. Vasc Surg. 49: 443-454.

[58] Swedenborg J, Eriksson P (2006) The intraluminal thrombus as a source of proteolytic activity. Ann. NY Acad. Sci. 1085: 133-138. doi: 10.1196/annals.1383.044.

[59] Vorp DA, Lee PC, Wang DH, et al (2001) Association of intraluminal thrombus in abdominal aortic aneurysm with local hypoxia and wall weakening. J. Vasc. Surg. 34: 291-299. doi: 10.1067/mva.2001.114813.

[60] Biasetti J, Gasser TC, Auer M, et al (2009) hemodynamics conditions of the normal aorta compared to fusiform and saccular abdominal aortic aneurysm with emphasize on thrombus formation. Ann. Biomed. Eng. 38: 380-390. doi: 10.1007/s10439-009-9843-6.

[61] Georgakarakos E, Ioannou CV, Volanis S et al (2009) The influence of intraluminal thrombus on abdominal aortic aneurysm wall stress. Int. Angiol. 28: 325-333.

[62] Bluestein D, Dumont K, De Beule M et al (2009) Intraluminal thrombus and risk of rupture in patient specific abdominal aortic aneurysm-FSI modeling. Compt. Meth. Biomech Eng. 12: 73-81.

[63] Georgakarakos E, Ioannou CV, Papahaliraou Y et al (2011) Computational evaluation of aortic aneurysm rupture risk: What have we learned so far?. J. EndovascTher. 18: 214-225. doi: http://dx.doi.org/10.1583/10-3244.1.

[64] Doyle BJ, Corbett TJ, Callanan A (2009) An experimental and numerical comparison of the rupture locations of an abdominal aortic aneurysm. J. Endovasc. Ther. 16: 322-335.

[65] Darling RC, Messina CR, Brewster DC, et al (1977) Autopsy study of unoperated abdominal aortic aneurysm. The case for early resection.Circulation. 56 (3 suppl): II 161-164.

[66] Soudah E, Vilalta G, Vilalta JA et al (2012) Idealized abdominal aortic aneurysm (AAA) geometry as predictor of hemodynamic stresses. Accepted for oral presentation in 6thEuropean Congress on Computational Methods in Applied Sciences and Engineering (ECOMAS 2012). Vienna Sep 10-14, 2012.

[67] Raghavan ML, Harbaugh RE (2005) Quantified aneurysm shape and rupture risk. J. Neurosurg. 102: 355-362.

[68] McGloughlin TM Doyle BJ (2010) New approaches to abdominal aortic aneurysm rupture risk assessment: engineering insight with clinical gain. Aterioscler. Thromb. Vasc. Biol. 30: 1687-1694.

[69] VandeGeest JP, Wang DHJ, Bohra A, Marakoun MS, Vorp DA (2006) A biomechanics-based rupture potential index for abdominal aortic aneurysm risk assessment. Ann. N.Y. Acad. Sci. 1085: 11-21.

[70] Li Z, Kleinstreuer C (2005) A new wall stress equation for aneurysm rupture prediction. An. of Biomedical Eng. 33: 209-213.

[71] Inzoli F, Boschetti F, Zappa M, Longo T, Fumero R (1993) Biomechanical factors in abdominal aortic aneurysm rupture. Eur. J. of Vasc. Surg. 7: 732-739.

[72] Mower WR, Buraff LJ, Sneyd J (1993) Stress distribution in vascular aneurysm: factors affecting risk of aneurysm rupture. J. of Surgical Research. 55: 1556-161.

[73] Vorp DA, Raghavan ML, Webster MW (1998) Stress distribution in aortic abdominal aneurysm: influence of diameter and symmetry. J. of Vasc Surg. 27: 632-639.

[74] He CM, Roach MR (1994) The composition and mechanical properties of abdominal aortic aneurysms. J. of Biomech Eng. 109: 298-304.

[75] Raghavan ML, Webster MW, Vorp DA (1996) Ex-vivo biomechanical behavior of abdominal aortic aneurysm: assessment using a new mathematical model. Ann Biomed Eng. 24: 573-582.

[76] Heng MS, Fagan MJ, Collier JW, Desai G, McCollum PT, Chetter IC (2008) Peak wall stress measurement in elective and acute abdominal aortic aneurysms. J. of Vasc Surg. 47: 17-22.

[77] González A, García de la Figal J (2009) Analysis of mechanical behavior of aorta section (in Spanish). IngenieríaMecánica. 12: 9-18.

[78] De Putter S, Wolters BJBM, Rutten MCM, Breeuwer M, Gerritsen FA, Van de Vosse FN (2007) Patient-specific initial wall stress in abdominal aortic aneurysm with a backward incremental method. J. of Biomech. 40: 1081-1090.

[79] Volokh KY, Vorp DA (2008) A model of growth and rupture of abdominal aortic aneurysm. J. of Biomech; 41: 1015-1021.

[80] Tong P, Fung YC (1976) The Stress-Strain Relationship for the Skin. J. of Biomech. 9: 649-657.

[81] Rodríguez JF, Ruiz C, Doblaré M, Holzapfel GA (2008) Mechanical stresses in abdominal aortic aneurysm: influence of diameter, asymmetry, and material anisotropy. J. of Biomech Eng. 130: 256-267.

[82] Holzapfel GA, Gasser TC, Ogden RW (2000) A new constitutive framework for arterial wall mechanics and a comparative study of material models. J. of Elasticity. 61: 1-48.

[83] Papaharilaou Y, Ekaterinaris J A. Manousaki E, Katsamouris AN (2007) A decoupled fluid structure approach for estimating wall stress in abdominal aortic aneurysms. J. of Biomech. 40: 367-377.

[84] Vorp DA, VandeGeest JP (2005) Biomechanical determinants of abdominal aortic aneurysm rupture. Arteriosclerosis, Thrombosis and Vascular Biology. 25: 1558-1566.

[85] Vascops Vascular diagnostics. On-line survey: Clinical assessment of AAA rupture risk. Are biomechanical predictors needed? (2007). Last access: Sept-15-2010. Available in: http://www.vascops.com/files/survey2006.pdf. Accessed: 2011 March 24.

Chapter 6

Abdominal Aortic Aneurysm in Different Races Epidemiologic Features and Morphologic-Clinical Implications Evaluated by CT Aortography

Ana Mladenovic, Zeljko Markovic, Sandra Grujicic-Sipetic and Hideki Hyodoh

Additional information is available at the end of the chapter

1. Introduction

By definition AAA is dilatation in diameter of the main arterial vessel in abdomen-abdominal aorta for over 50% compared to expected normal diameter (1). This dilatation is caused by gradual decrease in elasticity and consistence of aortic wall, usually including weakness in middle layer of aortic wall (tunica media), which leads to extension of extern layer (tunica adventitia) and/or inner layer (tunica intima) (2,3). Blood that is pumped through aorta under pressure, gradually stretches this weakened wall and most often creates aneurysmatic dilatation.

The disease is most often found in elderly population (4). In 5% of population older than 65, presence of AAA is confirmed (4,5). It has been noticed that this disease is about 6 times more frequent in males than in female population (6).

Over time, most of AAA (around 80%) increases in diameter (2,6). It is not possible to foresee which aneurysm will increase and which one will remain stable. In most cases, the growth of aneurysm is slow. Aneurysms measuring 5 or more cm in diameter increase for 4-8mm annually (7). Aneurysms with greatest diameter of 4-5 cm grow 3-7mm annually, while those smaller than 4 cm in diameter grow 2-5 mm on average (7,8). This long-term disease presents with nonspecific symptoms and is often unpredictable. The most frequent complication and leading cause of mortality (over 80%) in patients with AAA is rupture.

In many epidemiologic studies it has been noticed that persons with positive family anamnesis for this disease, have significantly higher risk of developing the aneurysm and its rupture. Furthermore, other risk factors for aneurysm have been identified, such as obesity, hypertension, smoking and elevated blood cholesterol level (9-14). The role od diabetes mellitus, which is a well known risk factor in development of occlusive disease of blood vessels, in terms of aneurysm development remains controversial (15-20).

There are two current therapeutic approaches. The first one is surgery and the other is endovascular (Endovascular Aortic Repair – EVAR). In about half of the patients with intact aneurysm, as well as in those with ruptured one, endovascular approach can be applied. Advantages of endovasular treatment are avoiding general anesthesia, laparotomy and clamping the aorta. The procedure lasts shorter and recovery is fast. However, there are some disadvantages or technical limitations of this procedure. It is not possible to place the graft if proximal neck of the anuerysm is smaller than 15mm and conical in shape (21,22), because origins of renal arteries could be covered. Also, the neck of the aneurysm should be orientated at the angle no smaller than 60º towards the sagittal plane of the aorta, iliac arteries must not be tortuous and must measure at least 9 mm in diameter (23,24). During relatively short period of clinical application and development of EVAR (from 1991) the problem of frequently inadequate commercially available aortic stent-grafts for yellow race and patients with low BMI (21) has arised. The appliation of EVAR in yellow race patients showed that only 23-42% grafts, with fabrically defined dimensions, are adequate, in 23-46% they need certain corrections, while in about 30% of patients there is a contraindication for stent placement (25,26,27,28). Contemporary experience in the application of EVAR showed that overall number of complications is relatively high, even up to 30-40%. Also, one of the reasons is a not precise enough preprocedural morphologic evaluation of AAA and early diagnostics of postprocedural complications.

Modern generations od multidetector CT units (generation 16 slice, 2004 to 64 slice detectors-2007), offered a new visualisation quality and possibility to obtain more relevant diagnostic information compared to DSA. MDCT aortography reaffirmed the significance of preprocedural evaluation which ensures obtaining numerous and high quality information in each and every situation, considering the place of graft insertion, graft design and overall indication for EVAR, as well as relevant postprocedural evaluation and early diagnstics of possible complications.

During last 3 years, MDCT units with 10-times lower exponential doses per examination were constructed (29-35). At the same time, routine use of high-resolution ultrasonography as non-ionizing morphologic imaging enabled screening programmes for AAA in elderly and high-risk populaton, that are conducted and in progress in many countries (36,37,38).

2. Body

Main hypotheses of this multicentric study are:

1. Positive family anamnesis for AAA, as well as trauma, personal history of diabetes mellitus and hypertension, smoking, elevated LDL cholesterol, which are risk-factors for AAA
2. There are significant anatomic-morphologic differences in aneurysmatic infrarenal aorta between Caucasian and Asian patients

Abdominal Aortic Aneurysm in Different Races Epidemiologic Features and Morphologic-Clinical
Implications Evaluated by CT Aortography

111

3. There are precise morphologic parameters based on MDCT aortography which determine indications and contraindications for EVAR, graft dimensions and the place of insertion
4. MDCT aortography enables early diagnostics of EVAR complications
5. The possibility of graft design in individual case is enabled by integrating measurements obtained by MDCT aortography in selective programme

The study was conducted in Clinical center of Serbia - Center for radiology and magnetic resonance and Institute for radiology, University Hospital Saporro (Japan), in period 2009-2011. In thiis study 31 Asian and 30 Caucasian patients with the infrarenal aortic aneurysm were included, as well as 130 Asian and 126 Caucasian patients with indication for CT aortography (CTA), which confirmed the absence of AAA. Election of patients of both races before referred to CT examination, was performed according to medical history, and definite indication for CT exam was set according to clinical findings and sonographic findings in distal aorta. Exclusion criteria were: rupture of aneurysm, aneurysm that exceeded infrarenal segment, discrete dilatation of aorta and finding of rough intramural and extraluminal calcifications in longer segment.

Data about risk factors for development of AAA (smoking, hypertension, elevated blood cholesterol level) were collected. One of the questions included the presence of diabetes mellitus in personal history. Questionnaire icluded demographic parameters (sex, age, race, education), antropometric data (body weight, body height, body surface, body mass index), personal history (diabetes, trauma, other) and family medical history (presence of AAA in relatives).

For classifying patients according to the level of nutrition, we used international classification recomended by World Health Organization (WHO) and US Institutes of Health: underweighted-BMI<18,4, normal weighted BMI between 18,5 and 24,9; overweighted BMI 25-29,9 and obese BMI>30. According to body height, all the patients were divided in 4 subgroups: shorter than 160 cm, between 160 cm and 170 cm, between 170-180 cm and taller than 180 cm.

Considering smoking, patients were divided into 3 subgroups according to duration of this habit: 10 years, between 10-20 years and over 20 years. Level of blood cholesterol over 3,4 mmol/l was considered elevated. For calculation of body surface (SA) we used Dubois & Dubois formula: SA= 0.20247 x height (m)0.725 x weight (kg)0.425. Considering that it is a complex logarithmic formula, we used software (calculator) for SA recommended by US National institutes of health (http://www.nih.gov). For the calculation of BMI we used established formula: BMI= body weight (kg) : body surface (m²).

3. 64-slice MDCT protocol and measurements used in the study

CTA examination in both centers was performed on the same CT unit of the same generation, type and model of the machine. We performed examinations on 64-slice VCT

Lightspeed unit (GE, Milwaukee, IL, US). In all cases we used non-ionic contrast agent in concentration of 320-370 (1 ml – 370 mg iodine) applied by automatic injector in cubital vein reaching flow rate of 5 ml/sec.

Taking into account heterogeneity of selected population by constitution, sex, race and age, and expected heterogeneity in „delay time" of the examination start, we used programme mode „SmartPrep" for defining the appropriate time, by selecting the spot in aorta where appearance of contrast agent triggers the acquisition. Helical mode was used in SmartPrep protocol, 120 kV, 250-700 mAs, rotation speed of the tube 0,35 with slice thickness of 1,25 mm with 64 slice detector in 0.625mm reconstruction.

Postprocessing was performed with the same selected applications in both centers:

Volume Viwer Analysis-CTA Aorta and   Advanced Vessel Analysis. Interobserver variability was avoided by the fact that examinations in both centers were performed by a single radiologist.

Number of global selected mathematic variables which define morphology at CTA examination usen in this study is 11. Overall number of methodologically defined transverse measurements is 36 (12 for infrarenal aorta and 24 for iliac arteries), overall number of linear measurements is 36 and volumetric measurements 3. All together, these measurements represent methodologic protocol used in the study for defining the morphology of aneurysmatic infrarenal aorta.

Linear, transverse and volumetric measurements were performed according to the protocol defined aforehead, which consisted of following parameters (Figure 1). All linear measurements were performed in 3 characteristic 2D and 3 characteristic 3D reconstructions (AP, PA and semi-oblique) and mean value was used as definite. We used software ruler tool which is a part of every Analysis-CTA Aorta. Proximal point for measuring aneurysmatic neck, linear distances of aorta, angle between AAA and all the other calculations were positioned in the orifice level of main renal artery. We performed following linear measurements:

- mean length of abdominal aorta (mm)(Figure 2)
- mean length of the neck of the aneurysm (mm)(Figure 3)
- mean linear distance from renal artery to aortic bifurcation (mm)(Figure 2)
- mean length of common iliac artery (mm)(Figure 4)
- AAA angle (degrees– °)(Figure 2)

Calculations of aortic and iliac arteries volumes represent a part of the basic package of Analysis-CTA Aorta programme. Start and end point are defined (Figure 1). Computer calculates only the lumen of blood vessel that contains contrast agent with no calcium deposits, and without wall structures in cases of thrombosed extraluminal mass; if AAA contains only the dilated vessel wall, the lumen is calculated in total.

Transverse measurements were performed using Advanced Vessel CT Aorta Analysis programme which enables linear differentiating the lumen of contrast agent that fills the vessel from intramural and endoluminal calcifications, considering the similar attenuation values of calcium and contrast agent which cannot be differentiated visually (there is a possibility of misinterpreting calcified plaque as vessel lumen). We performed 6 typical measurements in the same plane, for the lumen of circulating blood (total of 12 "flow" diameters)(F.d.) and 6 measurements in the same plane for diameters of circulating blood together with thrombosed blood, aneurysm content and thickness of the vessel wall (total of 12 „real"diameters)(R.d)(Figure 5, Figure 7).

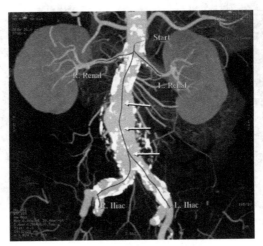

Figure 1. Characteristic points of interest to mark the CT angiographic analysis in Figure 2D.

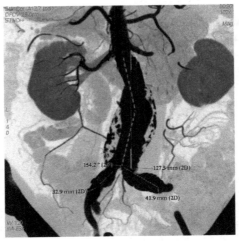

Figure 2. CT linear measurements of the aorta in the 2D image: mean length of abdominal aorta, mean linear distance from renal artery to aortic bifurcation and AAA angle

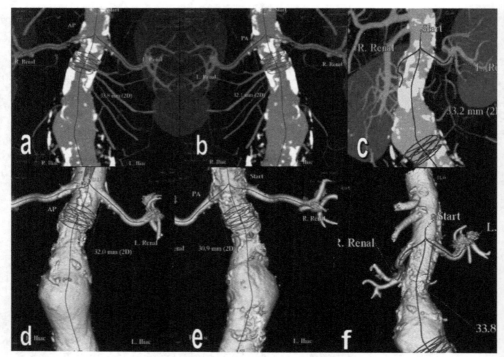

Figure 3. AAA neck length in 3 characteristic measurements in 2D (a-c) and 3D image (d-f).

The points of transverse measurements of abdominal aorta (a.a.) and common iliac artery (a.i.c.) performed in this study were following:

a.   infrarenal, in the level of the neck of the aneurysm, the largest and the smallest F.d. and R.d. (F.d.a.a 1, F.d. a.a 2, R.d. a.a 1 and R.d. a.a. 2)

b.   in the middle part of abdominal aorta, largest and the smallest F.d and R.d diameter (F.d. a.a 3, F.d. a.a 4, R.d. a.a 3 and R.d. a.a. 4)

c.   just above the aortic bifurcation, the largest and the smallest F.d and R.d diameter (F.d. a.a 5, F.d. a.a 6, R.d. a.a 5 and R.d. a.a. 6);

d.   proximal parts of both common iliac arteries distally from aortic bifurcation, the largest and the smallest F.d and R.d diameter (F.d. a.i.c 1, F.d. a.i.c 2, R.d. a.i.c 1 and R.d. a.i.c 2);

e.   middle parts of both common iliac arteries below aortic bifurcation, the largest and the smallest F.d and R.d diameter (F.d. a.i.c 3, F.d. a.i.c 4, R.d. a.i.c 3 and R.d. a.i.c 4);

f.   distal parts of both common iliac arteries above their bifurcations, the largest and the smallest F.d and R.d diameter (F.d. a.i.c 5, F.d. a.i.c 6, R.d. a.i.c 5 and R.d. a.i.c 6);

The precise localization of transverse measurements was defined according to the linear reconstruction of aorta and iliac arteries.

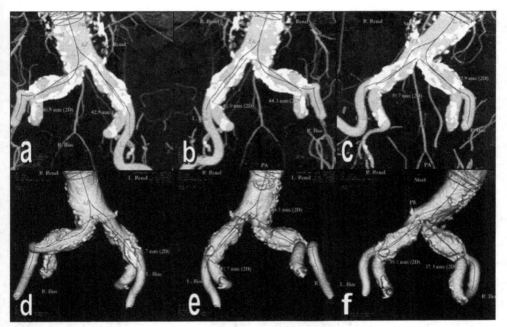

Figure 4. Measuring the length of the c.i.a in characteristic 3 position (AP, PA and oblique) in 2D (a-c) and 3D image (d-f)

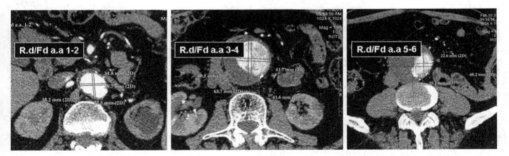

Figure 5. Transverse measurement of infrarenal aortic aneurysms (diameters Rd and Fd)

As a variable part of the protocol of morphologic measurements in this study, depending on the individual case, we performed other diagnostic explorations enabled by selected computer application, such as:

a.   Defining tissue structure (attenuation) in the region of interest (Figure 8)
b.   Defining the configuration of the blood vessel (Figure 9)
c.   Defining calcifications (Figure 10)
d.   Dynamic analysis of contrast agent flow
e.   MDCT aortoscopy (Figure 11)
f.   Coronal or sagittal 3D reconstruction (Figure 12)

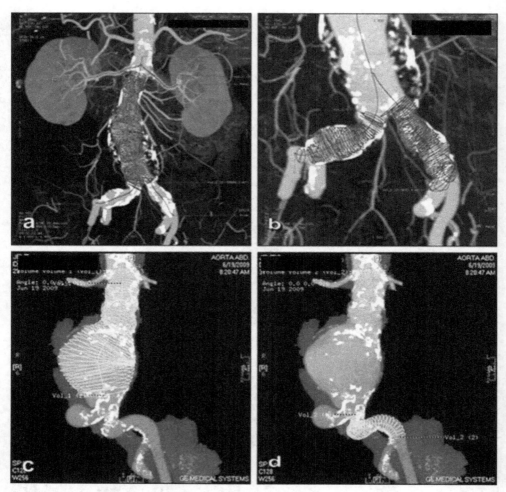

Figure 6. MD CT volumetric measurement of infrarenal aorta and aa.iliace comm bill in patients with calcium channel intraluminal nodular induration (a,b) patients with AAA and without calcium induration in the wall (c,d).

a) Defining tissue structure (attenuation) in the region of interest in different planes (most often transverse and sagittal). Using this exploration, known as „color mapping" it is possible to determine the density of the tissue in ROI or mean tissue density in the wider region. According to the attenuation distribution, it is possible to determine the structure or density of thrombotic aneurysmatic blood as well as differentiate contrast agent from calcified plaques which are pointed intraluminally. Every color represents a range of some interval of tissue density from 20-800 HU. Contrast agent is always represent by color green, low-density strustures (thrombus, blood, fat) by blue, atherosclerotic deposits by yellow and calcified indurations by red.

Abdominal Aortic Aneurysm in Different Races Epidemiologic Features and Morphologic-Clinical
Implications Evaluated by CT Aortography

117

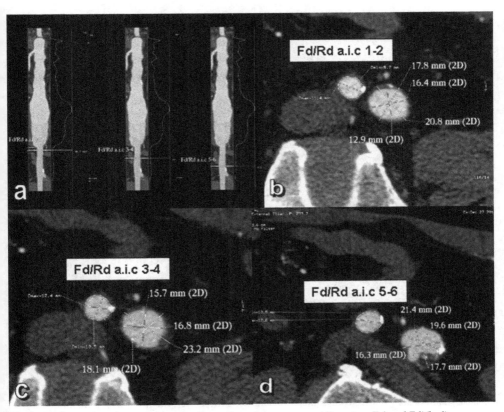

Figure 7. Transverse measurement of infrarenal aortic aneurysms (diameters Rd and Fd)(b-d)
compared to the linear angiographic image (a) (a)

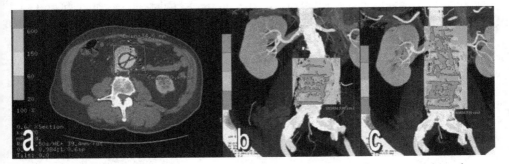

Figure 8. Defining tissue structure (attenuation) in the region of interest in the transverse (a) and
coronary reconstruction (b,c)

b) Defining the configuration of the blood vessel enables precise visualization in cases of
suspected dissection of the vessel wall and enables defining the wall thickness in all planes.
Furthermore, it enables clear graphic demarcation of the lesions of aortic wall and

differentiating from the extraluminal lesions. Additional option is definition of calcified indurations inside the „contoured" picture.

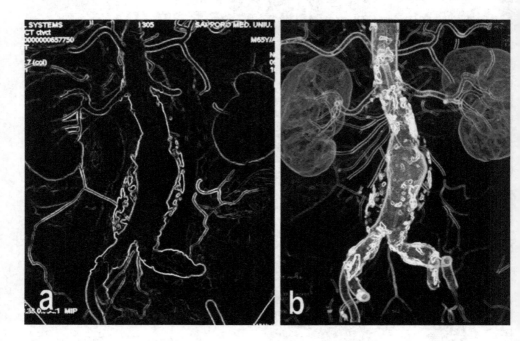

Figure 9. Contouring infrarenal aorta: linear (a) and with intramural calcifications (b)

c) Isolated defining extraluminal calcifications (Figure 3.21. a), intramural calcifications and altogether in frontal reconstruction along the aortic segment, in selected planes and positions. This exploration may imply on therapeutic approach in two projections at the level of c.i.a

d) Dynamic analysis of contrast agent flow represents the review of video-recording in selected plane, most often transverse or frontal, where dynamic of the contrast agent flow in aortic lumen can be analysed in real time mode.This exploration has a specific value in postprocedural evaluation and diagnostics of early complications of EVAR, most of all the proximal endoleak as a frequent complication. It is more sensitive than conventional digital aortography video -recording

e) MDCT aortoscopy, known also as „virtual aortography", is a special visualization option in „advanced" options of MD CT aortography, which is offered in standard postprocessing units of 16-64 slice MDCT units from the year 2007. It is a relatively simple, but powerful method of endoluminal examination in all planes, that enables optical presentation of the aortic wall inner surface, lesions of the aortic walls, the extent of anuerysmatic dilatation, endoluminal plaques and vessel arborization.

Abdominal Aortic Aneurysm in Different Races Epidemiologic Features and Morphologic-Clinical
Implications Evaluated by CT Aortography

119

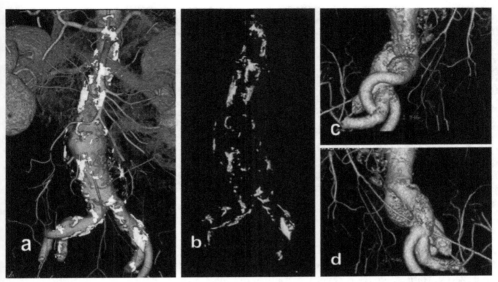

Figure 10. Defining calcifications of AAA - the level of the aortic extraluminarly (a) and intramural (b)

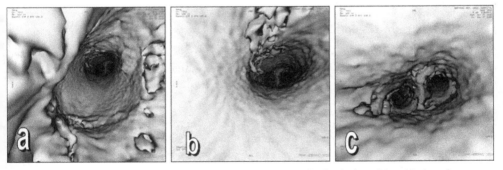

Figure 11. MDCT aortoscopy the level of renal arteries (a), middle third of a.a (b) and before the
bifurcation (c)

f) Coronal or sagittal 3D reconstruction (VR 3D cut). It is a postprocessing option from the
standard group which is more often used in diagnostics of parenchymatous organs and
heart, and represents „listing" slices at selected distance (0,625 mm at least) in 3D
presentation of the organ or lesion. In AAA, it can be used for visualization of thrombotic
mass and its structure considering heterogeneity and the presence of calcified indurations.
The analysis can be preformed in 6 standard planes: AP – anteroposterior; PA –
posteroanterior; L –left lateral, R – right lateral, I – inferior-superior; S – superior-anterior,
and additionally in every non-standard plane of rotated 3D image, which defines 4D
visualization in terms of movement.

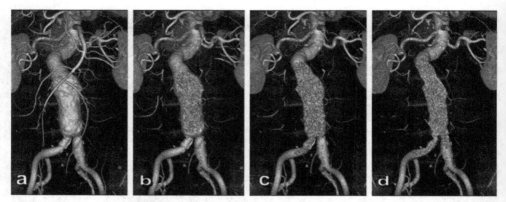

Figure 12.VR 3D cut option in coronary reconstuction in the antero-posterior direction (a) in 3 planes (b,c,d)

4. Statistic methodology

Considering the heterogeneity of the population included, as well as the number of analyzed variables, we used several statistical models for data analysis in this study:

Univariant and multivariant staistical methods – for testing statistic significance of difference between parameters for qualitative variables, as well as quantitative variables, univariant methods were used

χ^2 test –for testing the relationship between non-parametric variabes.

ANOVA - one-sample analysis of variance- univariant analysis of the effect of one selected factor on dependent variable. Comparing mean values, standard deviations in development of aneurysm between races and in the same race compared to control subjects, was performed using this method.

Median Test, Kolmogorov-Smirnov Z-test analysis of the mutual influence (of the selected variable among the groups), testing the compatibility of controls and patients in terms of developing the aneurysm, between races, and in the same race compared to the controls.

We determined the correlation coefficient (Pearson correlation) related to groups, smoking habit, and smoking history of all the subjects included, subjects according to sex (in males and females seperately).

According to univariant logistic regression analysis (ULRA) we tested the influence of selected variable (risk factors) and their correlation on the aneurysm development at the probability level $p \leq 0,01$.

Regression analysis (logistic model) In the model of MLRA we included all variables (risk factors) that were confirmed by univariant logistic regression analysis (ULRA) to be connected to the aneurysm development at the level of $p \leq 0,01$, so we determined the independent risk factors for development of aneurysm in all the subjects, and then seperately for male and female groups. All the variables were additionally tested in terms of age.

Odds Ratio (OR) or (expB) with confidence interval of 95%- chance ratio, or the possibility of the selected happening, the assessment of the correlation of risk factors (happening) and disease occurrence (development of aneurysm).

Statistic significance was determined at the level of probability of the null hypothesis p ≤ 0.05 to p<0.0001. Statistical analysis was performed using SPSS ver.20, while graphs and tables were edited using MICROSOFT OFFICE (EXCEL and WORD).

5. Study results

Distribution of patients according to the site of aneurysm, mean values ± SD in demographic and anthropological criteria and CT measurements between two races of the respondents suffering from AAA is shown in Table 1. The other criteria did not find statistically significant differences in relation to race in patients with AAA.

Demographic / Anthropological variables, MD CT measurements	AP with AAA Mean±Std.Dev.	EP with AAA Mean±Std.Dev.	ANOVA, F	p
age	75,60±6,13	61,13±10,97	39,75	0,001***
hight (cm)	159,90±8,85	176,63±8,20	57,70	0,001***
body weight (kg)	56,46±11,55	80,00±11,99	59,94	0,001***
surface area (m2)	1,58±0,18	1,97±,189	70,50	0,001***
BMI (kg/m2)	22,04±3,77	25,38±3,19	13,64	0,001***
aneurysm neck length	22,73±6,9	38,72±11,92	3,176	0,013**
aver.c.i.a.length	47,41±12,99	59,68±15,25	11,25	0,001***
aver.distance a.a.	84,39±31,58	63,27±50,76	3,65	0,05*
Fd-a.a1	19,05±3,95	22,87±6,44	7,65	0,01**
Fd-a.a2	22,08±4,13	26,88±7,62	9,22	0,001***
Rd-a.a1	24,06±4,98	29,39±9,28	7,67	0,01**
Rd-a.a2	26,18±5,79	31,57±10,98	5,66	0,02*
Rd-a.a3	32,53±12,37	43,42±20,74	6,11	0,02*
Rd-a.a4	34,46±12,75	48,07±22,35	8,39	0,01**
Rd-a.a6	28,91±10,90	36,61±17,29	4,25	0,04*
volume c.i.a.	6405,86±2819,07	8560,63±5145,87	4,05	0,05*

Table 1. Distribution of patients according to the site of aneurysm, mean values ± SD of age, height, body weight, surface area, BMI index, aneurysm neck length, aver.c.i.a.length, aver.distance a.a., Fd-a.a1, Fd-a.a2, Rd-a.a1, Rd-a.a2, Rd-a.a3, Rd-a.a4, Rd-a.a6 and volume c.i.a. - where the parameters are found statistical differences (*,**) and the difference is highly statistically differences (***).

Distribution of respondents to the AP and EP aneurysm and control groups the same race by age, gender, BMI and body height is shown in Table 2.

Age / Gender BMI, Body height		patients with aneurysm				patients without aneurysm			
		AP		EP		AP		EP	
		No	%	No	%	No	%	No	%
Age	≤ 74	13	41,90	26	86,60	62	47,69	114	90.47
	≥74	18	58,10	4	13,40	68	52,31	12	9,53
Gender	Male	25	83,3	24	77,4	58	46,03	90	83,3
	Female	5	16,7	7	22,6	68	53,97	40	16,7
BMI (kg/m^2)	< 18,4	0	0,00	3	9,68	3	2,38	7	5,38
	18,5 -24,9	12	40,00	22	70,97	96	76,19	113	86,92
	25-29,9	15	50,00	6	19,35	24	19,05	7	5,38
	> 30	3	10,00	0	0,00	3	2,38	3	2,31
Body height (cm)	< 160	14	45,20	0	0,00	73	56,15	0	0,00
	160-170	12	38,70	7	23,3	50	38,46	24	19,05
	≥171	5	16,10	14	46,70	7	5,38	73	57,94
Total		31	100	30	100	126	100	130	100

Age χ^2=13,322; p=0,0001
Gender χ^2=0,337; p=0,561
BMI χ^2=12,785; p<0,005
Body height χ^2=28,57; p<0,0001

Table 2. Distribution of respondents to the AP and EP aneurysm and control groups the same race by age, gender, BMI and body height.

The presence of factors in patients and control subjects as well as univariant regression analysis (ULRA) for assessment risk-factors among patients and controls in AP and EP groups of patients is shown in Table 3a. The presence of risk-factors in patients and control subjects as well as multinivariant regression analysis (MLRA) for assessment risk-factors among patients and controls in AP and group of patients is shown in Table 3b and the presence of risk-factors in patients and control subjects as well as multinivariant regression analysis (MLRA) for assessment risk-factors among patients and controls in EP group of patients is shown in Table 3c.

PREDICTORS	AP patients with aneurysm		EP patients with aneurysm	
	Unst.B	*p	Unst.B	*p
(Constant)	9,549	0,000	27,901	0,000
Age (up to and over 75 years)	-0,096	0,848	0,912	0,591
Height (< 160, 160-170, ≥171 cm)	-0,050	0,896	0,657	0,382
BMI (< 18,4, 18,5-24,9, 25-29,9, > 30)	0,466	0,351	-3,386	0,000
Smoking (yes/no)	3,254	0,000	1,348	0,496
Smoking (to10,10-20, over 20 years)	-2,284	0,000	-2,969	0,001
BP (>140/90) (yes/no)	-1,695	0,003	-2,725	0,009
LDL- cholesterol (>3,4 mmol/l) (yes/no)	-4,677	0,000	-4,545	0,000
Diabetes Melitus (yes/no)	3,238	0,000	3,121	0,011

Tab 3a

* p value according to the results ULRA (p ≤ 0,01)

PREDICTORS		OR	95% confidence interval	*p
Smoking	no	0,069	0,005-0,874	0,003
	yes			
Length of smoking (years)	to 10	7,608	2,836-20,408	0,0001
	10-20			
	over 20			
Hypertension (> 140/90)	no	3,831	1,079-10,911	0,037
	yes			
LDL- cholesterol (>3,4 mmol/l)	no	11,817	3,734-37,396	0,0001
	yes			

Tab 3b

* p value according to the results of MLRA

PREDICTORS		OR	95% confidence interval	*p
BMI	< 18,4	4,923	1,873-12,941	0,001
	18,5-24,9			
	25-29,9			
	> 30			
Length of smoking (years)	to 10	2,784	1,743-4,446	0,0001
	10-20			
	over 20			
Hypertension (> 140/90)	no	3,421	1,089-10,767	0,036
	yes			
LDL- cholesterol (>3,4 mmol/l)	no	6,696	2,092-21,430	0,001
	yes			

Tab 3c

* p value according to the results of MLRA

Table 3. The presence of risk-factors in patients and control subjects as well as multinivariant regression analysis (MLRA) for assessment risk-factors among patients and controls in EP group of patients.

6. Evaluation of the metodology of imaging studies

Generation of spiral CT units enabled the examination of large blood vessels for the first time as a substitute for the invasive conventional angiography, most importantly for aorta, extracranial arteries of the neck and skull base, main trunks of visceral arteries of thorax and abdomen and ilio-popliteal vessels. There have been numerous attempts to affirm spiral angiography for the exploration of 2nd and 3rd order arteries of parenchymatous organs, but diagnostic sensitivity was disappointing (33,39). Development of CT technology from the year 2000, enabled the start of new epoch with multidetector CT units, that brought amazing possibilities of image acquisition and spatial to temporal resolution ratio (30,31). In the same terms, a new postprocessing editing of transverse CT images was developed, offering faster, more detailed and accurate reconstruction possibilities in all planes. Definitely, MDCT examination established itself as diagnostically most sensitive in postprocedural evaluation of AAA and became method of choice in this field. In year 2007, exponential dose for the examination of infrarenal aorta using standard protocol at 64-slice unit, was approximatelly 6-8 mSv for both sexes. In obese patients it was somewhat higher (29). During the following 3 years, introducing new pulse generators and faster rotating tubes in clinical practice, exponential dose for CT exam of infrarenal aorta was lowered for 8-10 times, remaining the preoccupation of inovators until now.

7. Evaluation of demographic, antropologic and epidemiologic results of the study

In the discussion of the results of this study, we used every available data base, but most of all US National Library of Medicine National Institutes of Health (www.ncbi.nlm.nih.gov/pubmed), as well as other browsers for medical papers in MEDLINE and other indexed publications. Browsing bibliographic data was performed using relevant key words (races, aorta, CT, aortography, MDCT, aneurysm etc.)

Sex distribution in both groups of patients and controls in this study showed three basic features: there is no statistically significant difference in terms of sex in patients, that in control Caucasian subjects predominant group consisted of females and that in analyzed groups of patients predomination of males was statistically significant. Compared to the most cited epidemiologic studies considering the sex of patients, showing 4-6 times more frequent development of aneurysms in men, in this study we showed slight predominance of male patients in Caucasian group (around 72%), while in Asian group the number of male patients was smaller (around 50%). According to available data on the frequency of AAA in different races, it is generally accepted that the disease is most frequent in Caucasian population (12,14). In USA, for example, the incidence of AAA is significantly higher in white males than Afro-americans, while in female population, there is no statistically significant difference in the occurrence of the disease. Asian population (yellow race) is the least frequently affected by AAA (10,12). In Africa, aneurysm of thoracic aorta is more frequent, as well as in Carribean population. African males are three times less affected than Europeans (40). Interesting epidemiologic fact might be that in Britain, the morbidity ratio of Asian population is insignificantly lower than Caucasians, which is not applicable for non-emigrants (9). In China, AAA is a rare disease, as well as in population of Indonesia (9).

It remains unclear why AAA predominantly affects male population. Almost all the studies that tangle this question, insist on the fact that male population has higher incidence of etiopathogenetic risk factors: arteriosclerosis, smoking, hypertension and elevated blood cholesterol level. Generally speaking, the cause of this fact remains unclear, and as predisposing factors arise hormones, genetic disposition, disposition to atherosclerosis, more frequent risk factors or the combination of aforementioned factors. Singh K and Bønaa KH from famous University Hospital of Tromsø, Norway, in their study including 6.386 subjest of both sexes, established the diagnosis of AAA using sonographic screening , in 263 (8.9%) males and 74 (2.2%) females (9,20). Bearing in mind that subjects ranged in age (form 24-85 years), they compared the diameter of infrarenal aorta in terms of age and concluded that in male population there was a progressive growth in diameter of infrarenal aorta during the process of ageing. The effect of elevated plasma fibrinogen level in male population also remained unclear (8,11,44).

In terms of age distribution, Caucasian patients are statistically significantly younger than Asian patients (for 15 years). Compared to other studies, European patients are shown to be significantly younger than in other Caucasian populations (21,40). This data becomes interesting if we analyze distribution by age subgroups, where dominant incidence in white race population is found in the subgroup of patients younger than 64 (66%), while almost half of these patients are even younger than 54. The same distribution is shown in the control group of this population. On the other hand, in the Asian group of patients, AAA occurs in much older population- dominant incidence was found in the subgroup of older than 75 (54,8%). In the light of these results, we can analyze AAA as a primary disease (in white race) or in the setting of generalized atherosclerotic pathologic changes in the process of ageing (yellow race). Special attention must be paid to EVAR procedure in the group of elderly population, patients with cardiopulmonary and cerebrovascular insufficiency.

Definite conclusion is that the incidence of AAA increases with age, which is explained by prolonged impact of risk factors, long period between latency of risk factors and aneurysm development, and increased sensitivity of aorta to risk factors in the process of ageing. Hypothetically, changes in elastin structure cause increased mechanic stress on collagen which forms a strong fiber network. Experiment models of aneurysmatic blood vessels showed that isolated destruction of elastin led to dilatation of the vessel for 25-65%; also, following dilatation and possible rupture occur due to the alteration of collagen (6). Half-life of elastin is considered to be 75 years, and aorta of adult does not have the ability to produce functional elastin (6,7,42).

In terms of correlation patient height in study population and control groups, we obtained expected results. There is a statistically significant difference in the average height (Caucasian population is 17 cm taller than Asian population, dominant group in Asian population are patients shorter than 160 cm, while in Caucasians dominant group consists of patients over 171 cm)(17,29).

Further, there is statistically significant difference in body weight in study populations-European patients weigh 25.6 kg more than the Asian population, on average. This might be explained by obesity as a modern social-medicine phenomenon in developed countries where there is an increase in AAA incidence. Body weight in this study arised as statistically significant risk factor for the development of AAA.

Considering the level of nutrition, in the yellow race the dominant group consisted of normal weighted (70,97%), while there was no obese subjects (with BMI over 30) in this population. On the other hand, in the white race population over 50% patients were overweighted and obese. BMI can be observed as a universal parameter nondependent of the race, and obtain valid results with the use of simple statistical models (21). This parameter excludes race constitutional features and heterogeneity of the subjects in terms of body weight and body height, since last two parameters in 20% of observed patients and control subjects showed no statistically significant difference. If we use BMI value of 23 (approximate height of 170cm and weight of 58kg-mean BMI value in both groups of patients BMI=22,04±3,77 for Asian group and BMI=25,38±3,19 for Caucasian group) as observation criterion, instead of race, and divide all the subjects in two subgroups, BMI-1 (BMI<23) and BMI-2 (BMI>23), a correlation of antropologic and morphologic parameters calculated by MDCT aortography can be obtained (21).

In this study, there was no statistically significant difference in the presence of risk factors in subjects of both groups. In the Asian population, only 3,2% showed no risk factors present, while in the Caucasian population this percentage was 3,3%. Since patients with no risk factors present represent statistically insignificant subgroup in both populations, we can consider the presence of risk factors as a leading impact factor on the pathogenesis of the development of AAA. Considering the number of present risk factors, in Caucasian population the dominant group consists of patient with 3 or 4 risk factors (40% + 30% = 70%), while in Asian population dominant group consists of patients with 2 or 3 risk facotrs present (45,2% + 19,4% = 64,6%). In terms of the presence and number of RF in patients of both races, there is statistically significant difference in development of the disease. In Asian population, AAA occurs most frequently in patients with 2 RF (with 1 or 2 RF: 64,6%) while in white race this percentage is almost 3 times lower, only 23,3%. As a conclusion, Asian population seems to be more prone to the development of this disease.

The number of associated risk factors in patients of Asian population is statistically significantly higher than in control subjects of the same population. Over 40% (41,54%) control subjects in this population showed no risk factors present, while 25,3% showed only 1 RF present. Number of subjects with 3 associated RF is insignificant (2,3%), while there were no subjects with all 4 RF present. In total, there was statistically significant difference in the presence of risk factors in the patients and controls of the Asian population. In the same term, there is a positive correlation in the presence of risk factors in the patients and controls in European population also, while it is especially applicable for the presence of 3 or 4 associated risk factors.

Abdominal Aortic Aneurysm in Different Races Epidemiologic Features and Morphologic-Clinical
Implications Evaluated by CT Aortography

127

Tha analysis of the results considering smoking as risk factor in all the study subjects independently of race and smoking history, there was statistically significant number of smokers in both subgroups of patients compared to controls. The analysis of the results considering male and female populations showed that in patients of both populations smoking represents an extremely significant risk factor for the development of AAA. The results of multivariant logistic regresssion analysis were concordant.

On the contrary, hypertension as a risk factor in this study was proven to be controversial. In both races, the number of patients with hypertension was not significantly different than the number of normotensive patients. Epidemiologically significant finding was that in Asian population the number of normotensive patients was for 17% higher than hypertensive, while in European population there was 20% more hypertensive than normotensive patients. Generally speaking, in patients of both populations, hypertension is more commonly found than in control subjects, especially in the European population.

One of the referring studies considering pathogenesis of peripheral vascular diseases (McConathy, Oklahoma Medical Research Foundation) showed that in AAA, the level of cholesterol in plasma is lower than in patients with stenotic-occlusive arterial diseases, as well as VLDL level and apolipoprotein B, C-III and E. Total cholesterol is shown to be a stastically significant factor in the study of Reed-a et al. performed in integrated clinical-autopsy study in the 20-year period on 8000 men living in Hawaii (9). This study predominantly addressed the question of atherosclerosis as a risk risk factor in the development of AAA. The results concordant to this study were obtained in the Whitehall study of Strachan, published in British Journal of Surgery in 2005 considering younger population. Integrated epidemiologic study included 18.403 men, aged 40-64, working as accountants, in the period of 18 years. There were 99 lethal cases of ruptured AAA, and smoking and elevated systolic presure were isolated. Considering type of cholesterol, LDL and less importantly VLDL, are considered the dominant risk factor by many previous studies on this subject.

The analysis of results considering diabetes melitus (DM) as a risk factor in this study showed some unexpected results. The first „paradoxal" finding was extremely low number of patients in both groups with DM (3 patients in each group), with no significant difference between groups. In control groups of both populations, the incidence of DM is lower than 30%, with no statistically significant difference between controls and patients in both poulations. The unexpected result is that higher incidence of DM is found not in patient, but in control group of both populations. The most stunning result is the correlation of the presence of DM in patients and controls of the white race, where disease is significantly more frequent in the control subjects. These results raise the question: Does DM have etiopathogenetic correlation with the development of AAA, or closer to the results of this study- is DM some kind of protective factor in the AAA development? Meta analysis of 11 relevant studies considering correlation of DM and etiopathogenesis of AAA shed light to this „paradox". Out of 11, 4 studies were excluded for no existing or inadequate control group. The rest of the studies showed that there is a small possibility of associated DM in patients with AAA (OR=0.65, 0.60-0.70, p<0.001)(30). 3 referring studies found decreased prevalence of DM in patients with AAA (17,18,20).

8. Evaluation of morphologic measurements

European population showed statistically significantly longer neck of the aneurysm. With the premise that the length of the neck of 15 mm is the minimal infrarenal distance needed for graft insertion, this study showed that 31,7% patients in the Asian populaion had contraindication for EVAR, e. g. length of the neck of the AAA shorter than 15 mm. Furthermore, the mean length of the anuerysmatic neck in this population is 18,49 mm. Analyzing the subgroup of the Asian population with the neck length < 15 mm, we found that in 8 of 11 patients this length was < 10 mm, 9 mm on average.

The neck of AAA is the place of the proximal insertion of the graft, and in most cases there is a small distance between the normal and pathologic structures of aortic wall. The largest number of EVAR complications, of endoleak type, occur in this proximal part of graft insertion (43). CT aortography (CT fluoroscopy), as a dynamic analysis, enables monitoring of contrast agent flow along the aorta, or the region of interest established in examination protocol. More accurately, due to small slice thickness (0,625 mm), high spatial and temporal resolution, possibility of retroreconstruction in postprocessing at the distance of 0,2 mm and other technical features of this exam, it is possible to analyze CT exam as continuous video-recording in various visualization extensions. Also, „film" can be stoppped and paused in every moment to analyze the segment in 3D and 4D projetions, in all planes and projections.

Valuable advantage of these possibilities is that aorta, AAA and graft can be evaluated in all morphologic features, from the lateral aspects and also as ortogonally isolated transverse projections, a feature which cannot be performed using conventional aortography. These visualization possibilities favour MDCT over conventional aortography or catheter aortography. Beside the fact that it is a non-invasive procedure, additional advantage is that more diagnostic information on the early complications, such as proximal endoleak, can be obtained. Exceptional software features in standard postprocessing alow measuring of the contrast flow rate above the insertion place, inside the graft and distally, as well as different features of AAA before theraputic procedure. Critical moment for the development of proximal endoleak is physical contact of the contrast (blood) with graft contours. As it advances in cranio-caudal direction, contrast flow rate changes as a function of age, constitutional and hemodynamic cardiovascular parameters (stroke volume, width of aorta, degree of sclerotic changes, tortuosity, dilatation, etc.), but usually varies in range of 20-40 cm/sec. If the length of AAA neck is at the critical value (10-20 cm) this contact occurs in the place where vessel wall is already weakened, and its contractility, elasticity and histology are changed. Proximal endoleak can occur anywhere in the upper circumference of the graft, can be minimal, discrete and without clinical manifestations. Also, it can remain minimal in a long period of time, but usually there is a certain degree of progression, dilatation and degradation of the graft function.

Abdominal Aortic Aneurysm in Different Races Epidemiologic Features and Morphologic-Clinical
Implications Evaluated by CT Aortography

129

Due to physical contact and strike of contrast flow onto the upper edge of the graft, the speed with which blood continues to flow, decreases gradually. Presumption is that the velocity gradient directly influences the possibility of proximal endoleak occurrence. Developing this hypothesis, in the sense of possible clinical implications and technical advances, study offered the idea that the first contact of contrast and graft occurs suprarenally, e. g. 2-3 cm cranially of the insertion place. As a consequence, in last 10 years, fenestrated grafts with suprarenal insertions have become comercially available (44,45). In this tudy, a new design of graft for AAA treatment is proposed, for patients with short aneurysmatic neck. Inovation is the annular extension of existing graft that is continuous with the basic graft on the back side, while it is opened on the front and lateral sides, where is also the orifice of renal arteries. If the force of contrast stroke at MDCT exam is marked as F1 in the common concept of insertion place, and as F2 in the proposed graft design with suprarenal insertion, we could say that F2>F1 and that blood, distally from the suprarenal insertion flows continuously with lower speed (29).

The angle between aneurysm and sagittal plane of aorta in Asian population was significantly larger than in Caucasian. Also, in Asian population there were no patients with contraindication for EVAR (considering mean angle and standard deviation), while in Caucasian population, this number was not statistically significant.

On the contrary to the length of infrarenal aorta, a.i.c. in control group of Caucasian population was statistically significantly longer than in Asian. The mean length of both femoral arteries in white race population was about 14 mm higher than in yellow race, which was statistically significant. There was no significant difference in the length of infrarenal aorta between Asian and Caucasian population, but the linear distance between lower renal artery and bifurcation was significantly higher in European patient group (mean value was about 20 mm longer). This result can be explained by variations in the angle of AAA. Compared to the Hong Kong authors, this study found that linear distance in the white race patients was twice longer (40).

Transverse CT measurements considering flow diameter were performed in advanced CT aortography postprocessing programme, after transverse visualizations in graphic tool „X-section". This software tool enables contouring flow diameter along complete length and is used for differentiating contrast agent from intraluminal and intramural calcifications, while it enables continuity and accuracy in measuring in each segment.

There was significant difference between the study populations at the level of largest and smallest flow diameter below main trunks of renal arteries (F.d. a.a. 1-2) as well as total diameter of aneurysm with the vessel wall structures at the level of maximum width of aneurysm (R.d. a.a. 3-4). Especially significant was the difference between diameters R.d. a.a. 3-4. To the best of our knowledge, there are no similar results published in literature, nor have these measurements been performed in populations of different races. CT aortographic measurements performed in this study were inspired by problems that doctors who perform EVAR encountered due to incompatibility of the comercially available grafts for the patients of yellow race.

Infrarenal segment of aorta in patients with AAA is a nondilated part. However, the fact that infrarenal segment of aorta in all the subject of Asian population was significantly wider than transverse diameter of control subjects, and additionally, that it is related to the neck which is not dialated in transverse diameter, leads to conclusion that AAA patients in general have wider aneurysmatic neck than infarenal segment of control subjects (with discrete aortic dilatation or normal findings). Furthermore, the width of this segment may be disposing factor for the development of AAA or/and vice versa, that the development of AAA leads to dilatation of the aneurysmatic neck.

Most of the studies showed that the diameter of abominal aorta aneurysm grows for 0,08 cm annually, so the most accurate conclusions could be obtained by comparing subjects of the same age (29,40).

Asian population with the presence of aneurysm had significanty higher following diameters F.d. a.i.c. 2-6 i R-d. a.i.c. 1-6. compared to controls, while in F.d. a.i.c 1 there was no significant difference. The most prominent result was found in the transverse diameters F.d. a.c.i 1 of patients and controls. This was the only parameter where there was no difference in patients and controls of the Asian population, while in Caucasian there was a border-line difference. The exact place is just above the bifurcation, where depending on the bifurcation angle, there is a different flow gradient that correlates with the angle of bifurcation, which is lower in the population of yellow race. Additionally, there is a subtle difference between the blood flow velocity of the aorta and proximal parts of iliac arteries. The changes in the vessel wall, as well as propagation of the aneurysm from aorta to iliac arteries, have no direct impact on Fd diameter.

9. Possibilities of computer integration in postprocedural evaluation of AAA

In the preprocedural evaluation of EVAR method, nowadays the use of separate workstation is common. It is often used by vascular surgeons in order to obtain 3D visualization and measuring in individual case, for precise planning and choice of suitable type and dimensions of the graft. Actually, they use specially developed software applications on Windows platform, which are suitable for personal computers; widely spread are „3Mensio surgery", "TeraRecon" and "OsiriX".

This study showed that there is clearly defined user's need to upgrade MDCT aortography postprocessing and integrate it with softwares alowing typization and individualization of stent grafts in each case, as a definite preprocedural finding, similar to stenting procedures in non-vascular interventional radiology.

10. Conclusion

This study showed that modern imaging techniques, particularly high-resolution MDCT diagnositcs, discovered fresh and unexpected possibilities to obtain new knowledge on anatomy and morphology of the human body, as well as numerous clinical implications, applicable to all organs, organic systems, pathologic and pathophysiologic features, and studies in the field of anatomy.

The use of modern low-dose MDCT diagnostics will allow the development of screening programmes for many diseases of enormous diagnostic significance, related to blood vessels, such as coronary disease, cerebrovascular insuficiency, arteriosclerosis etc. In conclusion, the possibilities of correlating anatomy and morphology of different races in the context of a particular disease or planned study are limitless with use of CT diagnostics.

Author details

Ana Mladenovic* and Zeljko Markovic
Faculty of Medicine Belgrade University, Clinical Center of Serbia, Center of Radiology and Magnetic Resonance, Serbia

Sandra Grujicic-Sipetic
Institute of Epidemiology Faculty of Medicine Belgrade University, Serbia

Hideki Hyodoh
Department of Radiology, Sapporo Medical University, Sapporo, Japan

Acknowledgments

Edition of this chapter is supported by GE Healthcare - Technopharm, Belgrade, Serbia.

11. References

[1] Ernst CB (1993) Abdominal aortic aneurysm. N Engl J Med. 328:1167–1172

[2] Dalen JE. (1983) Diseases of the aorta. In: Petersdorf RG, Adams RD, Braunwald E, et al., eds. Harrison's principles of internal medicine. 10th ed. New York, NY: McGraw-Hill Book Company. pp.1488-91.

[3] Thompson RW, Geraghty PJ, Lee JK (2002) Abdominal aortic aneurysms: Basic mechanisms and clinical implications. Curr Probl Surg. 39(2):110–230.

[4] Beckman JA (2006) Aortic aneurysms: pathophysiology, epidemiology, and prognosis .In: Creager MA , Dzau VJ , Loscalzo J , eds. Vascular Medicine . Philadelphia:Saunders Elsevier, Inc . pp. 543 – 559.

[5] Tilson MD, Gandhi RH (1995) Arterial aneurysms: etiological considerations. In: Rutherford RB, ed. Vascular surgery. 4th ed. Philadelphia, PA: WB Saunders Company. pp. 253-64.

[6] Anidjar S, Kieffer E. (1992) Pathogenesis of acquired aneurysms of the abdominal aorta. Ann Vase Surg. 6:298-305.

[7] Patel MI, Hardman DT, Fisher CM, et al. 1995) Current views on the pathogenesis of abdominal aortic aneurysms. J Am Coll, Surg. 181:371-82.

---

* Corresponding Author

[8] Dobrin PB. (1989) Pathophysiology and pathogenesis of aortic aneurysms: current concepts. Surg Clin North Am 69: 687-703.

[9] James F. Blanchard (1999) Epidemiology of Abdominal Aortic Aneurysms, Epidemiologic Reviews by The Johns Hopkins University School of Hygiene and Public Health. Vol. 21, No. 2

[10] Stephen W.K. Cheng, Albert C.W. Ting and Simon H.Y. Tsang (2003) Epidemiology and Outcome of Aortic Aneurysms in Hong Kong, World Journal of Surgery. 2, 241-245.

[11] Yii MK. (2003) Epidemiology of abdominal aortic aneurysm in an Asian population. Source, ANZ J Surgery 73(6):393-5.

[12] Spark JI, Baker JL, Vowden P, Wilkinson D. Source (2001) Epidemiology of abdominal aortic aneurysms in the Asian community. Br J Surg. 88(3):382-4.

[13] Vowden P, Wilkinson D. (2001) Epidemiology of abdominal aortic aneurysms in the Asian community. Br J Surg. 88(3):382-4.

[14] Wei WI, Siu KF, Wong J. (1985) Abdominal aortic aneurysm in Chinese patients. Br J Surg. 72(11):900-2.

[15] Oxlund H, Rasmussen LM, Andreassen TT. (1989) Increased aortic stiffness in patients with type 1 (insulin-dependent) diabetes mellitus. Diabetologia 32:748-52.

[16] Forouhi NG, Merrick D, Goyder E, Ferguson BA, Abbas J,Lachowycz K. (2006) Diabetes prevalence in England, 2001 estimates from an epidemiological model. Diabet Med. 23(2):189-97.

[17] Wild S, Roglic G, Green A, Sicree R, King H. (2004)Global prevalence of diabetes: estimates for the year 2000 and projections for 2030. Diabetes Care. 27(5):1047-53.

[18] Ubink-Veltmaat LJ, Bilo HJ, Groenier KH, Houweling ST, Rischen RO, Meyboom-de Jong B. (2003) Prevalence, incidence and mortality of type 2 diabetes mellitus revisited: a prospective population-based study in The Netherlands (ZODIAC-1). Eur J Epidemiol. 18(8):793-800

[19] Kang SS, Littooy FN, Gupta SR. (1999) Higher prevalence of abdominal aortic aneurysms in patients with carotid stenosis but without diabetes. Surg. 126:687–692.

[20] Popov Petar, Ružićić Dušan, Babić Srđan, Tanasković Slobodan, Gajin Predrag. Lozuk Branko, Radak Đorđe. (2011) Učestalost pojave aneurizme abdominalne aorte u bolesnika sa diabetes mellitusom, Medicinska istraživanja. 45:23-34.

[21] Ana S. Mladenovic, Zeljko Markovic, Hideki H Hyodoh, and Tatjana Stosic-Opincal. (2012) Correlation of CT Aortography Measurements of Infrarenal Aortic Aneurysms and Body Mass Index in Preprocedural Evaluation for Endovascular Repair, Clinical Anatomy. DOI 10.1002/ca.22027

[22] Stephen WK, Cheng, Albert CW, Ting, Pei Ho, Jensen T. P. (2004) Poon Aortic Aneurysm Morphology in Asians: Features Affecting Stent-Graft Application and Design. Journal of Endovascular Therapy. 6: 605-612.

[23] Cambria Richard P., LaMuraglie Glenn M., Gertler Jonathan P., Abbott William M., Waltman Arthur C. (2000) Endovascular Repair of Abdominal Aortic Aneurysm: Current Status and Future Directions, AJR: 175:332-343

[24] Ahn SS, Rutherford RB, Johnston KW. Reporting standards for infrarenal endovascular abdominal aortic aneurysm repair. J Vasc Surg. 1997;25:405-410.

[25] Carpenter JP, Baum RA, Barker CF, Golden MA, Mitchell ME, Velazquez OC, Fairman RM. (2001) Impact of exclusion criteria on patient selection for endovascular abdominal aortic anerysm repair. J Vasc Surg. 34:150-4.

[26] Parody JC, Palmaz JC, Barone HD. (1991) Transfemoral intraluminal graft implantation for abdominal aortic aneurysms. Ann Vasc Surg 5(6):491-499.

[27] MacSweeney ST, Powell JT, Greenhalgh RM. (1994) Pathogenesis of abdominal aortic aneurysm. Br J Surg 81:935-41.

[28] Lazar Davidović, Miroslav Marković, Dušan Kostić, Ilijas Činara, Dragan Marković, Živan Maksimović, Slobodan D. Cvetković, Radomor B. Sinđelić, Tanja Illc. Ruptured Abdominal Aortic Aneurysms: Factors Infl uencing Early Survival. Ann Vasc Surg. (2005) 19(1): 29-34.

[29] Ana S. Mladenovc, Zeljko Z. Markovic, Hideki H. Hyodoh, Sandra Grujicic-Sipetic, NakajimaYasuo. (2011) Quantification of Dilated InfrarenalAorta by 64 Multidetector Computed Tomographic Evaluationin Preventing EVAR Complications in Patients of Different Races, Journal of Computer Assisted Tomography. 35 462-467

[30] Hirose Y, Hamada S, Takamiya M. (1992) Aortic aneurysms: growth rates measured with CT. Radiology 185:249-52.

[31] Bellon EM, Miraldi FD, Wiesen EJ. (2004) Performance evaluation of computed tomography scanners using a phantom model. Am J Roentgenol;132:345-352.

[32] Rubin GD. (2001) Techniques for performing multidetector-row computed tomographic angiography. Tech Vasc Interv Radiol. 4: 2-14.

[33] Pamela T. Johnson, Jennifer K. Chen, Bart L Loeys, Harry C. Dietz, Elliot K. Fishman. (2007) MDCT Angiography Findings, AJR 2007;189:226.

[34] Flohr TG, Schaller S, Stierstorfer K, Bruder H, Ohnesorge BM, Schoepf UJ. (2005) Multi-Detector Row CT Systems and Image-Reconstruction Techniques, Radiology 235:756-773.

[35] Saini S. (2004) Multi-Detector Row CT: Principles and Practice for Abdominal Applications Radiology. 233:323-327.

[36] Lederle FA, Walker JM, Reinke DB. (1988) Selective screening for abdominal aortic aneurysms with physical examination and ultrasound. Arch Intern Med. 148:1753-6.

[37] Collin J, Araujo L, Walton J. (1988) Oxford screening programme for abdominal aortic aneurysm in men aged 65 to 74 years. Lancet. 2:613-15.

[38] Arko FR, Filis KA, Seidel SA. How many patients with infrarenal aneurysms are candidates for endovascular repair? (2004) The Northern California experience. J Endovasc Ther. 11:33–40.

[39] Brewster DC , Cronenwett JL. (2003) Guidelines for the treatment of abdominal aortic aneurysms. Report of a subcommittee of the Joint Council of the American Association for Vascular Surgery and Society for Vascular Surgery . J Vasc Surg. 37(5) :1106 – 17

[40] Ana S Mladenović, Zeljko Z Markovic, Hideki H Hyodoh. (2011) Anatomic differences of the distal aorta with dilatation or aneurysm between patients from Asia and Europe as seen on CT imaging. European Journal of Radiology, doi:10.1016/j.ejrad.2011.05.014

[41] Brewster DC, Cronenwett JL, Haller, Jr JW, Johnston KW, Krupski WC, Matsumura JS. (2003) Guidelines for the treatment of abdominal aortic aneurysm: report of a subcommittee of the Joint Council of the American Association for Vascular Surgery and Society for Vascular Surgery. J Vasc Surg 37:1106-1117

[42] Alcorn HG, Wolfson SK Jr, Sutton-Tyrrell K. (1996) Risk factors for abdominal aortic aneurysms in older adults enrolled in the Cardiovascular Health Study. Arterioscler Thromb Vase Biol. 16:963-70.

[43] Brewster DC , Cronenwett JL. (2003) Guidelines for the treatment of abdominal aortic aneurysms. Report of a subcommittee of the Joint Council of the American Association for Vascular Surgery and Society for Vascular Surgery . J Vasc Surg. 37 (5) :1106-17.

[44] Greenhalgh RM , Brown LC , Kwong GP , Powell JT , Thompson SG. (2004) EVAR trial participants. Comparison of endovascular aneurysm repair with open repair in patients with abdominal aortic aneurysm (EVAR trial 1), 30-day operative mortality results: randomised controlled trial . Lancet . 364: 843-8.

[45] Lazarus HM. (1992) Endovascular grafting for the treatment of abdominal aortic aneurysms. Surg Clin North Am 72:959–968.

Chapter 7

Studying the Flow Dynamics Within Endografts in Abdominal Aortic Aneurysms

Efstratios Georgakarakos, Antonios Xenakis, George S. Georgiadis,
Konstantinos C. Kapoulas, Evagelos Nikolopoulos and Miltos Lazarides

Additional information is available at the end of the chapter

1. Introduction

Endovascular Treatment (EVAR) is considered the treatment of choice for the majority of Abdominal Aortic Aneurysms (AAA) nowadays, since it demonstrates improved perioperative morbidity and aneurysm-related mortality, comparing to conventional open repair. However, despite the initial technical success and early discharge of the patient, this technique is amenable to early and late complications, the most important of which are the endoleaks (ie. recurrence of blood flow detection within the aneurysm sac) accompanied sometimes with variable degrees of intrasac pressurization (Georgakarakos et al, 2012a). Furthermore, the hemodynamic changes that the endograft sustains during the follow-up period make it prone to positional changes with subsequent risk for endograft migration and loss of sealing between the endograft and either the aneurysm neck or the iliac fixation sites.

Computer-enhanced geometric modeling and Finite Volume Analysis have been used to study the biomechanical behavior of the aortic aneurysms before and after the insertion of the endograft device (Georgakarakos et al, 2012b). Numerical modeling of endovascular-treated AAA is used to determine the stresses and forces developed on AAA sac and stent-graft materials in-vivo, estimating hemodynamic parameters, such as the pressure and stress distribution over the main body, the bifurcation, the limbs of a stent-graft or the drag and displacement forces predisposing to graft migration. Consequently, the study of flow dynamics within aortic endografts holds a fundamental role in the delineation of the endograft behavior under pulsatile flow, providing useful information for developing and modifying the endograft design and surgical techniques. This chapter discusses the aforementioned changes, by using three-dimensional (3D) reconstructed endograft model.

2. Reconstruction of the AAA endograft model

Finite Volume Analysis technique has a crucial role in the computational research of hemodynamic systems, utilizing small subsections (elements) of 3-dimentional structures created by segmentation and meshing. By solving Navier-Stokes equations for all finite volumes of the model, Computational flow dynamics (CFD) techniques utilize numerical methods and algorithms to analyze problems that involve fluid flows. Furthermore, Fluid Structure Interaction (FSI) methods combine fluid and structural equations, solved either simultaneously or separately (partitioned approach), in order to determine the flow fields and solid body stresses on a deformable model. Most researchers acquire information on the 3D AAA realistic, complex geometry using patient-specific DICOM data derived from high-resolution spiral CT or MR angiography (Georgakarakos et al, 2012b).

Our study group used a reconstructed 3D model of a AAA endograft using commercially available appropriate, validated software (MIMICS 13.0, Materialise NV, Leuven, Belgium), based on the DICOM images derived from contrast-enhanced high-resolution computed tomography. The computational model (**Figure1**) includes the aortic neck proximal to the endograft and the iliac arteries distal to the endograft limbs. A validated Finite Volume analysis software ANSYS v 12.1 (Ansys Inc., Canonsburg, PA, USA) was used for Computational Fluid Dynamics (CFD). The velocity and pressure waveforms during a period of 1.2 s as previously described in a one-dimensional fluid-dynamics model for the abdominal aorta (Olufsen et al, 2000 and Li et al, 2005) were used for both models as inlet and outlet boundary conditions. Blood was assumed to be non-Newtonian fluid, according to the Carreau-Yasuda model, with a density of 1050 kg/m^3.

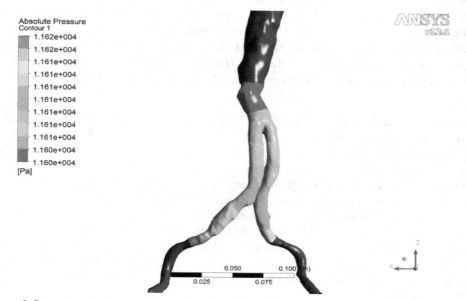

Figure 1. Reconstructed images of the aortic endograft using purpose-developed software.

Accordingly, the velocity streamlines and the pressure distribution were calculated over the entire surface of the endograft and are demonstrated in 6 distinct time-phases through the cardiac cycle (**Figure2**). For study reasons, the cardiac cycle was dived in six distinct phases, namely the late diastole (t_1), the accelerating systolic phase (t_2), the peak systolic phase (t_3), the late deceleration (t_4), the end-systolic (t_5) and the early diastolic phase (t_6).

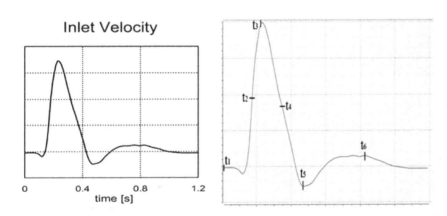

Figure 2. Plot of the flow waveform used for the calculations in our endograft model (left panel). Six distinct phases are depicted in each cardiac cycle. t_1 depicts the late diastole, t_2 the accelerating phase, t_3 represents the peak systolic phase, t_4 the late deceleration, t_5 depicts the end-systole and t_6 the early diastolic phase (right panel).

3. Changes in flow patterns and pressure distribution

Figures 3-8 depict the flow patterns in the endograft throughout the cardiac cycle. A flow disturbance is seen near the inlet zone (panel top-left) during the late diastole, t_1 (Figure 3). The flow pattern is normalized during the entire systolic phase, ie. t_2 to t_4 (Figures 4-6) and exhibits disturbance again, from the the end-systole t_5 early diastole t_6 (Figures 7,8). Interestingly, there is disturbed flow in the iliac limb unilaterally (left) during the decelerating systolic phase (Figure 6), whereas the irregular flow is also transmitted in the contralateral (right) iliac limb, during the next time-step (end-systolic phase, t_5, Figure 7).

	t_1	t_2	t_3	t_4	t_5	t_6
Pressure values (mmHg)						
Max	87	167	147	120	104	97
Min	87	136	136	115	102	96

Table 1. Maximum and minimum values of pressure in the endograft surface, for the different phases of the cardiac cycle. Excessively high values of pressure due to alteration in the iliac limbs geometry were excluded (outlier values).

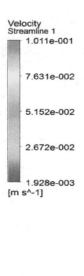

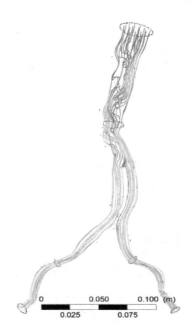

Figure 3. The velocity streamlines, as demonstrated for the late diastolic phase (t_1).

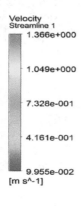

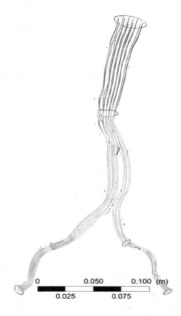

Figure 4. The velocity streamlines, as demonstrated for the accelerating systolic phase (t_2).

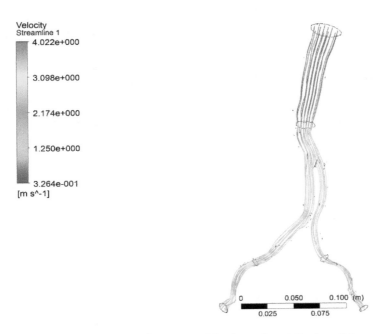

Figure 5. The velocity streamlines, as demonstrated for the peak systolic phase (t₃).

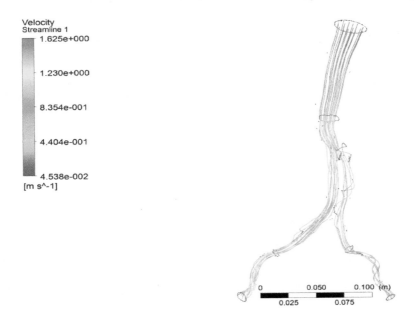

Figure 6. The velocity streamlines, as demonstrated for the decelerating systolic phase (t₄).

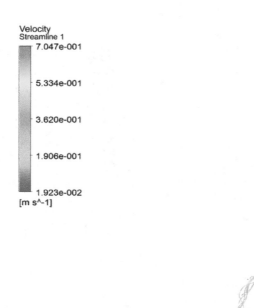

Figure 7. The velocity streamlines, as demonstrated for the end-systolic phase (t₅).

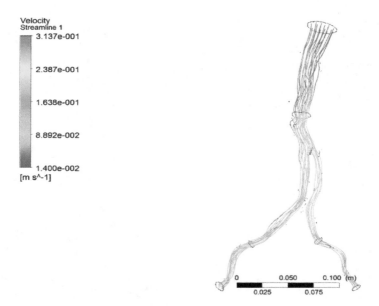

Figure 8. The velocity streamlines, as demonstrated for the early diastolic phase (t₆).

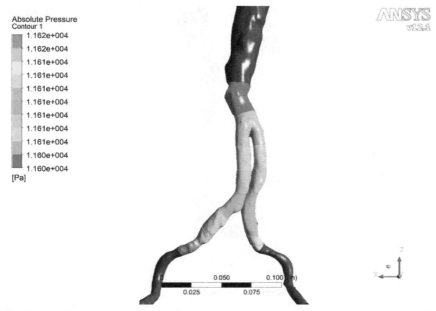

Figure 9. The distribution of pressures across the endograft, as demonstrated for the late diastolic phase (t_1).

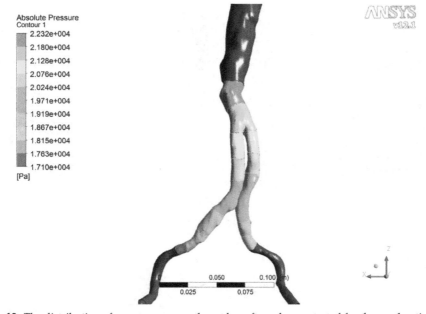

Figure 10. The distribution of pressures across the endograft, as demonstrated for the accelerating systolic phase (t_2).

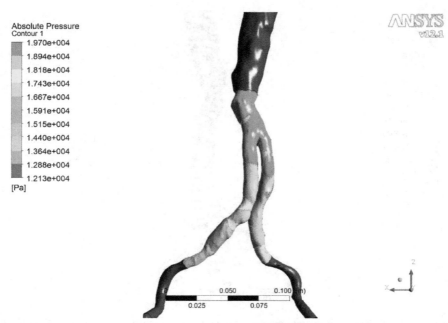

Figure 11. The distribution of pressures across the endograft, as demonstrated for the peak systolic phase (t_3).

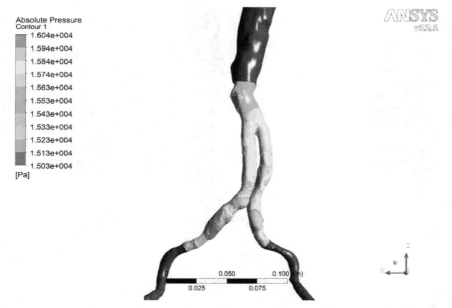

Figure 12. The distribution of pressures across the endograft, as demonstrated for the decelerating systolic phase (t_4).

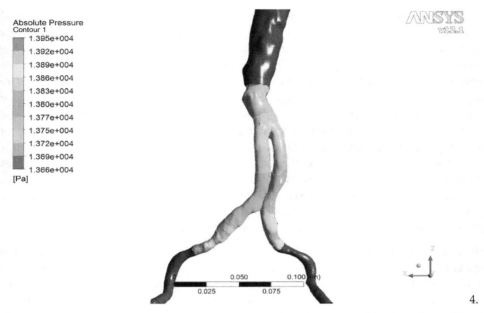

4.

Figure 13. The distribution of pressures across the endograft, as demonstrated for the end-systolic phase (t_5).

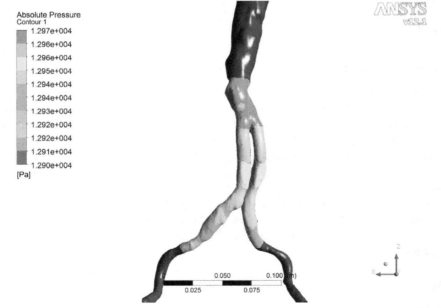

Figure 14. The distribution of pressures across the endograft, as demonstrated for the early diastolic phase (t_6).

Table 1 depicts the minimum and maximum pressure values along the endograft surface, for the different phases of the cardiac cycle (as described above). As depicted in Figures 9-14 and Table 1, there is a similar, homogenous distribution of the pressure values along the different parts of the endograft during the diastolic phase (t_6 and t_1). However, when it comes to the systolic phase (t_2 and t_4), there is a marked linear decrease of the pressure values from the endograft inlet to the iliac limbs (outlet). The greatest pressure value difference is marked in the accelerating systolic phase (t_2). Interestingly, the highest and lowest pressure values are demonstrated in the inlet-main body area and the iliac limbs of the endograft, respectively, during the accelerating and peak systolic phase, whereas this pressure relation is reversed in the decelerating systolic phase (t_4), where the highest values are located distally (outflow). Moreover, there seems to be a narrower range of pressure distribution in the peak systolic phase (t_3). Finally, in the early diastolic phase (t_6) there is again a reverse in the pressure distribution compared to the early systolic phase, with the highest pressure being located in the inflow area of the endograft.

Figures 15-17 demonstrate the vertical velocity patterns and the secondary flow fields in the different parts of the endograft, during the peak systolic and the diastolic phase. The bifurcation of the endograft in two distinct outflow tracts (iliac limbs) causes a disturbance of flow especially in the secondary flow fields and generation of local vortices mainly in the proximal iliac parts (Figure 16), before this marked difference is subsided in the most distal iliac outflow parts (Figure 17). This pattern is also met in the diastolic phase, but with a greater discrepancy being present in this phase (Figures 15-17). In both iliac limbs there was a skewing of the flow towards the inner wall and significant flow separation towards the outer wall.

4. The forces exerted on the endograft surface

The forces applied on the surface of the endograft are demonstrated in Figures 18-20. The forces generated by the pressure are directed mainly vertical to the endograft surface (Figure 18) throughout the cardiac cycle. The tangential forces are mainly caused by the flow of blood and the boundary layer that is formed near the aortic wall, while their direction is depended on the cardiac phase. So, their vector heads forward during the early, peak (Figure 19) and late systolic phase, whereas the direction is reversed during the end systole (Figures 2 and 20) and late diastole. Notably, the values of the tangential forces are lower than the pressure ones by many orders of magnitude. The total sum of the pressure and viscous forces acting on the surface of the graft resolving into the x, y and z components, determines the drag forces that the endograft is subjected to, making it prone to migration.

5. Discussion

(CFD) techniques provide a valuable and reliable tool in the study of the hemodynamic behavior of the cardiovascular system after therapeutic interventions (Frauenfelder, 2006).

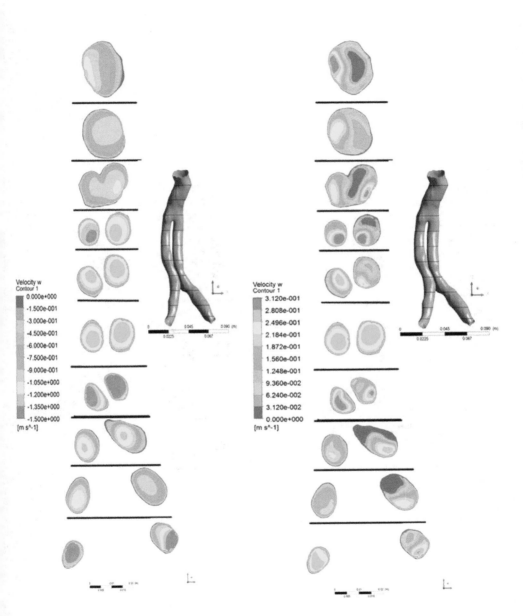

Figure 15. Distribution of velocity values in the transverse axis (-z) along ten cross-section of the endograft, during the peak systolic phase (left panel) and the diastolic phase (right panel).

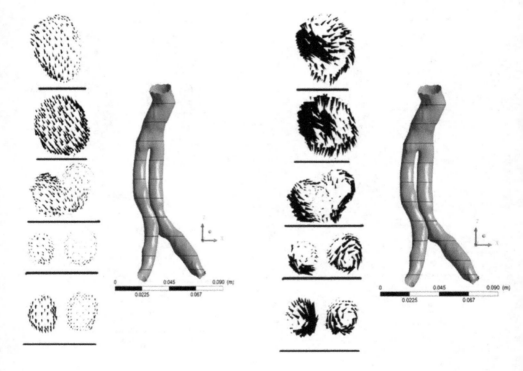

Figure 16. Distribution of velocity profiles in the secondary flow fields along the transverse axis (-z) in the 5 cephalad cross-sections (endograft inlet to proximal thirds of the iliac limbs) of the endograft, during the peak systolic (left panel) and the diastolic (right panel) phase.

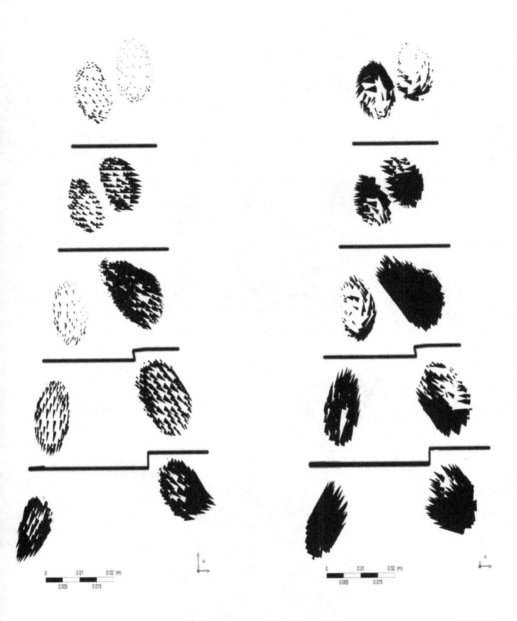

Figure 17. Distribution of velocity profiles in the secondary flow fields along the transverse axis (-z) in the 5 caudal cross-sections (proximal to distal thirds of the iliac limbs) of the endograft, during the peak systolic (left panel) and the diastolic (right panel) phase.

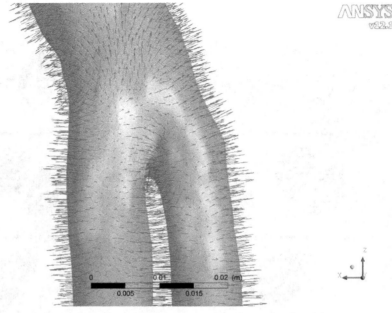

Figure 18. The pressure forces on the endograft bifurcation area (peak systolic phase).

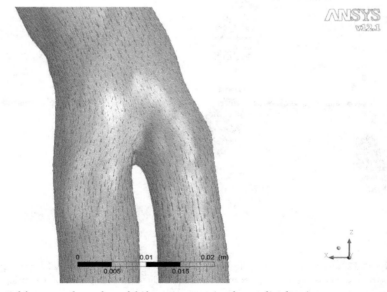

Figure 19. The tangential forces on the endograft bifurcation area (peak systolic phase).

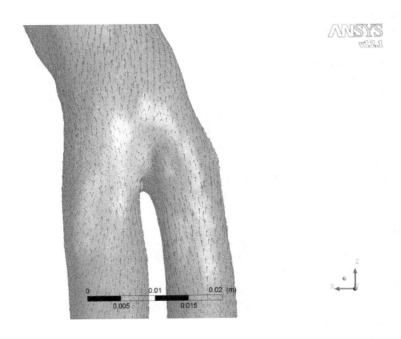

Figure 20. The tangential forces on the endograft bifurcation area during the end systolic phase, t$_5$).

The insertion of an endograft causes alterations in the hemodynamic environment of the AAA, regarding the pressures and stresses exerted on the AAA sac as well as the flow patterns inside the endograft lumen (Molony et al, 2009). There is a reduction in the intrasac pressure and the stress values on the sac of the stented AAA, leading to sac shrinkage. Chong and How (2004) used flow visualization and laser Doppler anemometry to study in vitro the flow patterns within a stent graft in different phases of the cardiac cycle. According to their study, the main trunk of the endograft is characterized by complex flow patterns with evidence of instability in systolic acceleration phase, developing into a number of vortical structures during systolic deceleration. The flow phenomena in the iliac limbs are strongly influenced by the geometry and the configuration of the limbs (Morris 2006 and Molony, 2008) and any degree of existing constriction caused in the iliac limbs. Basically, the flow in both limbs is triphasic, with a large retrograde component in end-systole (Chong and How, 2004) and formation of recirculating zones. The profiles are significantly more disturbed in the deceleration phase than at maximum velocity (Chong and How, 2004).

Finally, local geometric factors play a role in the determination of velocity values and flow patterns (recirculating zones, flow separation, skewed flow, vortices and Dean flows) with the out-of-plane endograft geometry determining greatly the outlet flow rates, flow patterns and drag forces (Morris 2006). Extrinsic constriction (due to calcified or stenosed iliac vessels) or excessive kinking in the iliac limbs can lead either to thrombosis of the graft limbs or altered flow patterns that induce excessive disturbances in shear stresses (not shown in our model), leading also to recirculating zones and prolonged transit times of platelets with consequent apposition and formation of thrombus in the endografts. The latter constitutes a rather common incidental finding, occurring more frequently that previously assumed (Wu et al, 2009). Finally, the study and understanding of the hemodynamic alterations and the parameters that influence them, could lead to better designs of endovascular grafts, in order to eliminate the factors that predispose to endograft migration as well as to generation of endoleaks (Figueroa 2009 and 2010, Liffman 2001, Mohan 2002).

6. Conclusion

Aortic endografts are subject to hemodynamic alterations that determine the flow patterns within the different parts of the endografts and influence the values and distribution of pressures and stresses onto their surface during the different phases of the cardiac cycle. Certain geometric factors such as the inlet-to-outlet ratio of the graft as well as the out-of-plane configuration of the main body and iliac limbs have been implicated as major determinants of the aforementioned hemodynamic alterations. Computational simulation techniques can help towards the understanding of these interactions and help us further design better endografts with greater resistance to migration, endoleaks and dislocation of modular stent-grafts, all of which are influenced by the hemodynamic environment that endografts are exposed to.

Author details

Efstratios Georgakarakos, George S. Georgiadis,
Konstantinos C. Kapoulas, Evagelos Nikolopoulos and Miltos Lazarides
"Democritus" University of Thrace Medical School, Alexandroupolis,
Greece

Antonios Xenakis
Fluids Section, School of Mechanical Engineering,
National Technical University of Athens, Athens,
Greece

7. References

Georgakarakos E, Georgiadis GS, Ioannou CV, Kapoulas KC, Trellopoulos G, Lazarides M. (2012a). Aneurysm sac shrinkage after endovascular treatment of the aorta: beyond sac pressure and endoleaks. *Vasc Med.*;17:168-73.

Georgakarakos E, Georgiadis GS, Xenakis A, Kapoulas KC, Lazarides MK, Tsangaris AS, Ioannou CV. (2012b). Application of bioengineering modalities in vascular research: evaluating the clinical gain. *Vasc Endovascular Surg.*;46:101-8.

Chong CK, How TV, Gilling-Smith GL, Harris PL. (2003). Modeling endoleaks and collateral reperfusion following endovascular AAA exclusion. *J Endovasc Ther.*;10:424-32.

Chong CK, How TV. (2004). Flow patterns in an endovascular stent-graft for abdominal aortic aneurysm repair. *J Biomech.*;37:89-97.

Figueroa CA, Taylor CA, Yeh V, Chiou AJ, Zarins CK. (2009). Effect of curvature on displacement forces acting on aortic endografts: a 3-dimensional computational analysis. *J Endovasc Ther.*;16:284-94.

Figueroa CA, Taylor CA, Yeh V, Chiou AJ, Gorrepati ML, Zarins CK (2010). Preliminary 3D computational analysis of the relationship between aortic displacement force and direction of endograft movement. J Vasc Surg.;51:1488-97.

Frauenfelder T, Lotfey M, Boehm T, Wildermuth S. (2006). Computational fluid dynamics: hemodynamic changes in abdominal aortic aneurysm after stent-graft implantation. Cardiovasc Intervent Radiol.;29:613-23.

Li Z, Kleinstreuer C, Farber M. (2005). Computational analysis of biomechanical contributors to possible endovascular graft failure. *Biomech Model Mechanobiol.*;4:221-34.

Liffman K, Lawrence-Brown MM, Semmens JB, Bui A, Rudman M, Hartley DE. (2001). Analytical modeling and numerical simulation of forces in an endoluminal graft. *J Endovasc Ther.*;8:358-71.

Mohan IV, Harris PL, Van Marrewijk CJ, Laheij RJ, How TV. (2002). Factors and forces influencing stent-graft migration after endovascular aortic aneurysm repair. *J Endovasc Ther.*;9:748-55

Molony DS, Callanan A, Morris LG, Doyle BJ, Walsh MT, McGloughlin TM. (2008). Geometrical enhancements for abdominal aortic stent-grafts. *J Endovasc Ther.*;15:518-29.

Molony DS, Callanan A, Kavanagh EG, Walsh MT, McGloughlin TM. (2009). Fluid-structure interaction of a patient-specific abdominal aortic aneurysm treated with an endovascular stent-graft. *Biomed Eng Online.*6;8:24.

Morris L, Delassus P, Grace P, Wallis F, Walsh M, McGloughlin T. (2006). Effects of flat, parabolic and realistic steady flow inlet profiles on idealised and realistic stent graft fits through Abdominal Aortic Aneurysms (AAA). *Med Eng Phys.*;28:19-26.

Olufsen MS, Peskin CS, Kim WY, Pedersen EM, Nadim A, Larsen J. (2000). Numerical simulation and experimental validation of blood flow in arteries with structured-tree outflow conditions. *Ann Biomed Eng.*; 28:1281-99.

Wu IH, Liang PC, Huang SC, Chi NS, Lin FY, Wang SS. (2009). The significance of endograft geometry on the incidence of intraprosthetic thrombus deposits after abdominal endovascular grafting. *Eur J Vasc Endovasc Surg.*;38:741-7.

Chapter 8

Splenic Artery Aneurysms

Ahmad Alsheikhly

Additional information is available at the end of the chapter

1. Introduction

The spleen is a wedge-shaped organ that lies in relation to the 9th and 11th ribs, located in the left upper quadrant of the abdomen (left hypochondrium), and partly in the epigastrium; thus, it is situated between the fundus of the stomach and the diaphragm (see the following image). The spleen is highly vascular and reddish purple; its size and weight are variable. Normally spleen is not palpable.

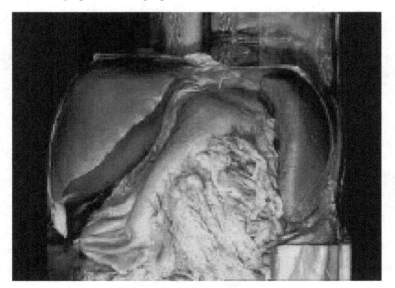

Figure 1.

The spleen develops in the cephalic part of dorsal mesogastrium (from its left layer; during the sixth week of intrauterine life) into a number of nodules that soon fuse to form a lobulated spleen. Notching of the superior border of the adult spleen is evidence of its multiple origins.[1]

The spleen has 2 ends, 3 borders, and 4 surfaces, as follows:

The 2 ends

The anterior end of the spleen is expanded and more like a border; it is directed forward and downward to reach the midaxillary line. The posterior end is rounded; it is directed upward and backward and rests on the upper pole of the left kidney.

The 3 borders

The superior border of the spleen is notched near the anterior end, the inferior border is rounded, and the intermediate border is directed toward the right.

The 2 surfaces

There are 2 surfaces: diaphragmatic and visceral. The diaphragmatic surface is smooth and convex. The visceral surface is irregular and concave and has impressions. The gastric impression is for the fundus of the stomach; this is the largest and most concave impression on the spleen. The renal impression is for the left kidney and lies between the inferior and intermediate borders. The colic impression is for the splenic flexure of the colon; its lower part is related to the phrenicocolic ligament. The pancreatic impression for the tail of the pancreas lies between the hilum and colic impression (see the image below).

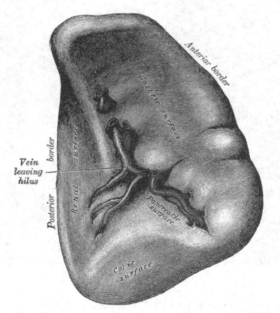

Figure 2. Spleen showing the different surfaces and impressions caused by different organs with relation to the hilum of the spleen.

1.1. Hilum

The hilum lies on the inferomedial part of the gastric impression. It transmits the splenic vessels and nerves and provides attachment to the gastrosplenic and splenorenal (lienorenal) ligaments.

1.2. Peritoneal relations

The spleen is surrounded by peritoneum and is suspended by multiple ligaments, as follows:

The gastrosplenic ligament: This ligament extends from the hilum of the spleen to the greater curvature of the stomach; it contains short gastric vessels and associated lymphatics and sympathetic nerves

The splenorenal ligament: This ligament extends from the hilum of the spleen to the anterior surface of the left kidney; it contains the tail of the pancreas and splenic vessels

The phrenicocolic ligament: This ligament is a horizontal fold of peritoneum extending from the splenic flexure of the colon to the diaphragm in the midaxillary line; it forms the upper end of the left paracolic gutter.

1.3. Visceral relations

The visceral surface of the spleen is related to the following organs:

- The fundus of the stomach
- Anterior surface of the left kidney
- Splenic flexure of the colon
- Tail of the pancreas

The diaphragmatic surface is related to the diaphragm, which separates the spleen from the pleura and the lung.

1.4. Blood supply

The blood supply of the spleen is by the splenic artery (in the past called the lienal artery), which is the largest branch of the celiac trunk. The artery passes through the splenorenal ligament to reach the hilum of the spleen. At the hilum, it divides into multiple branches. Within the spleen, it divides into straight vessels called penicillin, ellipsoids, and arterial capillaries.

The splenic circulation is adapted for the mechanism of separation and storage of the red blood cells. On the basis of the blood supply, the spleen has superior and inferior vascular segments. The 2 segments are separated by an avascular plane.

Apart from its terminal branches, the splenic artery gives off branches to the pancreas, 5-7 short gastric branches, and the left gastro-omental (gastroepiploic) artery (see the image below).

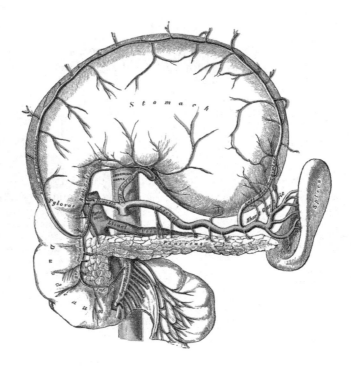

Figure 3.

1.5. Venous drainage

The principal venous drainage of the spleen is through the splenic vein. It is formed at the hilum and runs behind the pancreas then joins the superior mesenteric vein behind the neck of the pancreas to form the portal vein. Its tributaries are the short gastric, left gastro-omental, pancreatic, and inferior mesenteric veins.

1.6. Lymphatic drainage

Splenic tissue proper has no lymphatics. However, a few arise from the capsule and trabeculae and drain to the pancreaticosplenic lymph nodes.

1.7. Nerve supply

Sympathetic fibers are derived from the celiac plexus.[2, 3, 4]

1.8. Surface marking

The spleen is marked on the left side of the back with the long axis of the 10th rib. The upper border is marked along the upper border of the 9th rib; the lower border, along the 11th rib. The medial end lies 5 cm from the midline, and the lateral extension is to the midaxillary line.[5]

Microscopically, the spleen is made up of 4 components: (1) supporting tissue, (2) white pulp, (3) red pulp, and (4) vascular system.

Supporting tissue is fibroelastic and forms the capsule, coarse trabeculae, and a fine reticulum.

The white pulp consists of lymphatic nodules arranged around an eccentric arteriole called the Malpighian corpuscle.

The red pulp is formed by a collection of cells in the interstices of the reticulum, in between the sinusoids. The cell population includes all types of lymphocytes, blood cells, and fixed and free macrophages. The lymphocytes are freely transformed into plasma cells, which can produce large amounts of antibodies and immunoglobulins. The vascular system traverses the spleen and permeates it.[3]

2. Physiologyof the spleen

The spleen is a major hematopoietic organ containing approximately 25 percent of the total lymphoid mass of the body; and it is capable of supporting elements of the erythroid, myeloid, megakaryocytic, lymphoid, monocytic, and macrophagic (reticuloendothelial) systems. As such, it is important in the following situations:

2.1. Phagocytosis

Phagocytosis is one of the most important functions of the spleen. The spleen forms a component of the reticuloendothelial system. The splenic phagocytes include reticular cells, free macrophages of the red pulp, and modified reticular cells of the ellipsoids. The phagocytes present in the organ remove debris, old and effete red blood cells (RBCs), other blood cells, and microorganisms; thus, the splenic phagocytes filter the blood. Phagocytosis of circulating antigens initiates the humoral and cellular immune responses.

This function is most apparent when the spleen has been removed, since splenectomized patients are susceptible to bacterial sepsis, especially with encapsulated organisms.

2.2. Hematopoiesis

The spleen is an important hematopoietic organ during fetal life; lymphopoiesis continues throughout life. The manufactured lymphocytes take part in immune responses of the body. In the adult spleen, hematopoiesis can restart in certain diseases such as chronic myeloid leukemia and myelosclerosis.

2.3. Active immune responses

Following antigenic stimulation, increased lymphopoiesis for cellular responses and increased formation of plasma cells for humoral responses occurs.

2.4. Storage of erythrocytes

The RBCs are stored in the spleen. Approximately 8% of the circulating RBCs are present within the spleen. However, this function is seen well in animals than humans.[6]

3. Splenic Artery Aneurysms (SAAs)

3.1. General considerations

An arterial aneurysm is one of the most common vascular disorders causing morbidity and mortality in humans. It occurs in most arteries of the body and is especially common in the elderly. They have a variable sizes, shapes, and locations.

An aneurysm is defined as a permanent localized dilatation of an artery having at least a 50% increase in diameter compared to the expected normal arterial diameter, so clinicians should know the normal arterial diameters throughout the body to decide the presence or absence of an aneurysm. [7]

Splenic artery aneurysms are a type of splanchnic arteries aneurysm, although the later are rare but clinically very important vascular conditions. These interesting lesions have been recognized since more than 200 years. [8, 9]

Splanchnic artery aneurysms represent intra-abdominal aneurysms that are not part of the aorto-iliac system and include aneurysms of the celiac, superior and inferior mesenteric arteries with their branches.

Of all intra-abdominal aneurysms, only approximately 5% affect the splanchnic arteries. (10) In general population, their prevalence has been estimated to be varying from 0.1% to 2 %. [11]

The frequency of the anatomic distribution of the splanchnic arteries aneurysms is estimated to be the following:

1. Splenic artery aneurysms (SAAs), 60% (see the image below).
2. Hepatic artery, 20%
3. Superior mesenteric artery, 6%
4. Celiac artery, 4%
5. Gastric and gasrtoepiploic arteries, 4%
6. Jejunal, ileal, and colic arteries, 3%
7. Pancreaticoduodenal and pancreatic arteries, 2%
8. Gastroduodenal artery, less than 1.5%
9. Inferior mesenteric artery, less than 1%. (11)

3.2. Prevalence and epidemiology

SAAs are the most common of the splanchnic artery aneurysms and account for as many as 60% of all reported splanchnic aneurysms. They are recognized for their significant potential

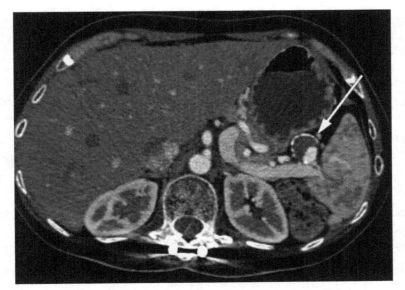

Figure 4. A Peripherally calcified, and thrombosed splenic artery aneurysm, (CT view)

to rupture. In spite of their relatively high prevalence in comparison to other splanchnic aneurysms, there are few large series in the literature. The prevalence of the lesion in the general population is low. A large general autopsy study estimated their all incidence to be 0.01 %(12), whereas more specific examination of the splenic arteries in an autopsy study of patients older than 60 years revealed an incidence of 10 %(13).

The prevalence of incidentally noted aneurysmal changes in the splenic artery on arteriographic studies was reported to be 0.78%, and such changes have been found incidentally in 0.1% to 10% of autopsies. (11).

In contrast to routine atherosclerotic or degenerative aneurismal diseases, SAAs are found much more commonly in women than in men with an approximate ratio of 4:1. (11), they are also noted to occur in younger patients at a mean age of 52 years. (14)

SAAs are usually saccular and less than 2 cm in diameter, with the majority being in the mid or distal portion of the splenic artery or at its bifurcation points. (14)

Giant SAAs with diameter larger than 10 cm have been reported, and in contrast to smaller SAAs, these lesions appear to be more common in men. (15)

3.3. Pathogenesis and aetiology

The most clinical risk factors are the following:

1.	Female gender.
2.	Multiple pregnancies.

3. Portal hypertension.
4. Systemic hypertension.
5. Arterial fibrodysplasia.
6. chronic inflammatory processes
7. Arteriosclerosis.
8. Less commonly, polyarteritis nodosa, systemic lupus erythematosus, and anomalous splenic artery origin. (16).

In one reported series, it was noted that 80% of the patients with SAAs were females who had an average of 4.5 pregnancies and 50% of females with SAAs had more than 6 pregnancies. (17, 18).

Portal hypertension may be present in 25% of patients with SAAs, while about 10% are awaiting liver transplantation. (19).

Blunt splenic trauma and pancreatitis frequently noted in association with SAAs. Local hemodynamic aspects, hormonal factors, and medial degeneration have all been considered as causative factors in the development of SAAs. (20).

Increased blood volume which results into increased cardiac output, and portal congestion are thought to be related to an increased splenic artery blood flow and SAAs formation. (21).

Impaired elastin formation and degeneration of the internal elastic lamina could be added as hormonal factors which contribute to SAAs formation during pregnancy; It seems that splenic artery is more susceptible to these changes than other vessels. (22).

Histological changes which are noted microscopically during SAAs formation include calcifications, intimal hyperplasia, arterial dysplasia, fibromuscular dysplasia, and medial degeneration. (23).

3.4. Clinical and diagnostic aspects of splenic artery aneurysms

Most SAAs are found incidentally at the time of first presentation during abdominal imaging examination for unrelated disorders. A classic calcified ring may be noted in the left upper abdominal quadrant on a plain x—ray film of the abdomen. (see the image below):

There may be an abdominal bruit, but the majority of cases are showing normal physical examinations especially with asymptomatic patients.

Symptoms are including the following:

1. Vague abdominal pain, nausea and vomiting.(24).
2. Symptoms related to compression of adjacent organs.
3. Sever left-sided pain due to rupture or acute aneurysm expansion.
4. Shock, abdominal distension, and death due to intraperitoneal rupture.
5. Double-rupture phenomenon which may occur in bout 20% to 30% of cases provides a proper diagnosis of rupture into the lesser sac, before free intraperitoneal rupture diagnosed.(25,26).
6. Gastrointestinal tract, pancreatic ducts, or splenic vein rupture.(27).

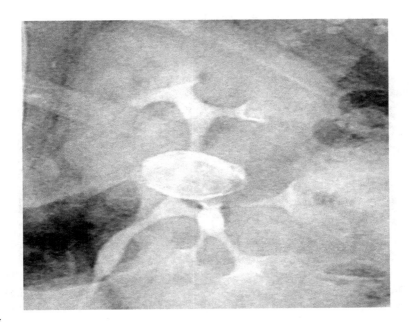

Figure 5.

The overall mortality of ruptured SAAs is about 25%.(26). Pregnancy may be associated with a rate of 20% to 50% of all ruptures.(28).

The association of SAAs and pregnancy is very well documented, in addition to that rupture during pregnancy usually occurs at the third trimester which can lead to maternal and fetal death of 80% to 90%, respectively.(29). Actually this can lead to understand the misdiagnosis of the situation as an obstetric emergency.

Rupture due to portal hypertension is associated with a rate of about 20% .(30).

3.5. Treatment of splenic artery aneurysms

Ruptured , symptomatic SAAs, and those in pregnant women require urgent treatment. Enlarging or those greater than 2 cm in diameter SAAs have less stringent indications, although these criteria are not absolute. Patients with portal hypertension or waiting for liver transplantation should be treated as well.(31). Patient's medical condition and age could play a role the treatment option. Most vascular surgeons would consider suitable elective intervention for asymptomatic patients with lesions those diameter is greater than 2 cm when the surgical risk is thought to be low. If one estimates the incidence of rupture to be 2% with a death rate of at least 25% when rupture has occurred, operative mortality rates should be less than 0.5% to justify elective surgical treatment, in one author's study.(31).

Traditional operative therapy of SAAs includes proximal and distal ligation or aneurysmectomy or both modalities for lesions in the proximal or middle part of the splenic artery.(see the images below).

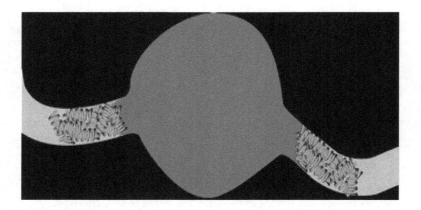

Figure 6. Drawing illustrates how coils are placed distal and then proximal to the aneurysm, thereby trapping the aneurysm and isolating it from the circulation, with resultant thrombosis of the aneurysm.

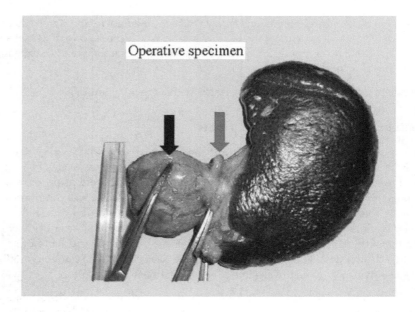

Figure 7.

Revascularization of the distal splenic artery in not generally warranted due to that collateral flow to the spleen in maintained by the short gastric arteries. For those lesions near to the splenic hilum, splenectomy is the most common procedure. Distal pancreatectomy may occasionally be needed for the treatment of these distal lesions as well. (24, 31, 32 and 33).

Laparoscopic repair of SAAs by clipping or exclusion has been reported; intraoperative ultrasonography is believed to be an important adjunct to this procedure.(34). Laparoscopic occlusion combined with coil embolization has been proposed as a treatment for aberrant SAAs located in the retropancreatic position, for which traditional procedures would be exceptionally difficult.(24,35).

Endovascular exclusion of SAAs has been used more recently with good success. Treatment options include coil embolization of the splenic artery both proximal and distal to the aneurysm itself, thereby effectively trapping the lesion. Other options include embolization of the aneurysm sac with coils or cyanoacrylate glue or both modalities simultaneously or occlusion of the lesion with percutaneous or open thrombin injection.(24,36). In addition, stent-grafting has been performed, especially for saccular lesions of the mid splenic artery. There has been some concern regarding splenic infarction and pancreatitis when embolization of very distal splenic artery lesions has been performed. (24, 37 and 38).

The objective of splenic arterial embolization is to improve the results of nonsurgical management. Indications for splenic arterial embolization vary, depending on local management protocols. embolization is performed with microcoils as distally as possible, to preserve perfusion to the splenic parenchyma. Patients with a high risk for secondary rupture of the aneurysm should undergo embolization with coils in a more proximal segment of the splenic artery to reduce the pressure in the splenic parenchyma and help the reservation of the spleen. The placement of coils in a middle segment of the splenic artery allows reconstitution of the blood supply through collateral vessels, principally via the short gastric and gastroepiploic arteries, to the patent distal splenic, transgastric, and transpancreatic arteries. Proximal embolization performed exclusively with coils decreases the volume of splenic arterial blood flow and thereby produces relative hypotension in the splenic bed, which allows the spleen to repair itself without infarction (39)

In a review of 48 endovascular procedures for splanchnic artery pseudoaneurysms, 20 interventions on the splenic artery were performed. Six end-organ infarcts were noticed, all were within the splenic bed. Two additional patients developed splenic atrophy diagnosed on CT scanning after previous embolization of the splenic artery, without clear clinical evidence of initial splenic infarction. (40). In another study, one episode of splenic infarction associated with sever pancreatitis was noted after embolization of a distal splenic artery aneurysm. (37). (see the image below).

Post-embolization transverse contrast-enhanced CT scan obtained at follow-up shows a coil within the splenic artery (arrow), as well as complete infarction of the spleen, which is not contrast enhanced.

However, other authors have reported splenic infarction after embolization of even more proximal SAAs as well. (41).

3.6. Results of different treatment options for splenic artery aneurysms:

The results of open operative therapy are dependent on whether the procedure is an elective or emergency one, in addition to the anatomical complexity of the lesion and the nature of the required repair. Elective procedures have significantly lower perioperative morbidity and mortality compared to the emergency techniques for ruptured aneurysms which carries death rate greater than 50% in many reported series. (42).

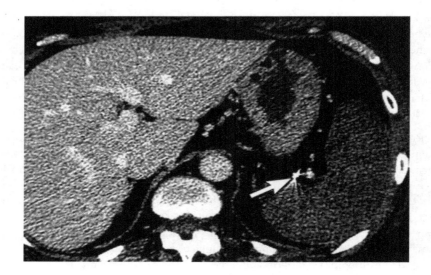

Figure 8.

Technical success after percutaneous coil embolization of SAAs is acceptable and ranges from 81% to 98%, although some studies showed that the presence of hemodynamic instability should not preclude endovascular management. (43,44).

End-organ ischaemia is an especial concern with regard to endovascular repair. Direct complications can result from this option of treatment such as arterial dissection, acute thrombosis, or embolization to nontarget tissues, or inadequate collateral circulation after deliberate vessel occlusion. It has been concluded that cases with aneurysmal lesion at the splenic hilum may be better managed by open repair and splenectomy.(45).

Although initial technical success rates with an endovascular procedure for treating SAAs approach 100%, the long-term success is less well defined.(46).

Ultrasound-guided percutaneous thrombin injection appears to be a viable method for treating failed endovascular interventions or even an alternative to initial endovascular treatment.(47). Actually, this technique is similar to thrombin injections for femoral artery pseudoaneurysms, were ultrasound or CT guidance or both are used to help delivering thrombin to the nidus of an aneurysm, thus facilitating thrombosis. This is particularly applicable to saccular aneurysms with a narrow neck arising from the parent vessel. Continued studies, even after secondary technical success, are imperative due to the natural history of SAAs after endovascular treatment remains unclear. This is true for saccular aneurysms treated by coil or thrombin embolization. Reports of reperfusion and even rupture after successful embolization support that a thrombosed aneurysm may not represent the definitive treatment in all cases.(47,48).

Author details

Ahmad Alsheikhly
Hamad Medical Corporation, Doha, Qatar

4. References

[1] Sadler TW. Chapter 14: Digestive system. In: *Langman's Medical Embryology*. 11th ed. Philadelphia, Pa: Lippincott Williams & Wilkins; 2009:215-6.

[2] Gray H. Chapter 88: The spleen. In: Standring S, ed. *Gray's Anatomy: The Anatomical Basis of Clinical Practice*. 39th ed. Edinburgh, UK: Churchill Livingstone Elsevier; 1239-44.

[3] Snell RS. Chapter 5: The abdomen: part II. The abdominal cavity. *Clinical Anatomy by Regions*. 8th ed. Baltimore, Md: Lippincott, Williams & Wilkins; 2007:259-60.

[4] Lee McGregor A, Decker GAG, du Plessis DJ. Chapter 8: The spleen. *Lee McGregor's Synopsis of Surgical Anatomy*. 12th ed. Oxford, UK: Butterworth-Heinemann; 1986:106-13.

[5] Romanes GJ. Abdomen: spleen. In: *Cunningham's Manual of Practical Anatomy. Vol II: Thorax and Abdomen*. Vol 2. 15th ed. New York, NY: Oxford Medical Publications, Oxford University Press; 1986.

[6] Guyton AC, Hall JE. Chapter 15: Vascular distensibility and functions of arterial and venous systems. *Guyton and Hall Textbook of Medical Physiology*. 11th ed. Philadelphia, Pa: Saunders; 2005:179-80.

[7] Johnston KW, Tilson MD, Stanley JC. The subcommittee on reporting standards for arterial aneurysm, International society for cardiovascular surgery. Suggested standards for reporting on arterial aneurysm. *J Vass Surg*, 1991; 13:452-458.

[8] Abbas MA, Stone WM, Bower TC, Panneton Jm, Cherry KJ. Splenic artery aneurysms: two decades experience at Mayo clinic. *Ann Vass Surg*. 2002; 16: 442-449.

[9] Carr SC Nemcek AA Jr, Yao JS. Current management of visceral artery aneurysms. *Surgery*. 1996; 120:627-634.

[10] Graham LM, Lindenauer SM. Celiac artery aneurysms: historic (1745- 1949) versus contemporary (1950-1984) differences in etiology and clinical importance. *J Vass Surg.* 1985; 2: 757- 764.

[11] Messina LM, Shanley CJ. Visceral artery aneurysms. *Surg Clin North AM.* 1997; 77:425-442.

[12] Moore SW, Guida PM, Schumacher HW: Splenic artery aneurysm. *Bull Soc Int Chir* 1970; 29:210-218.

[13] Bedford PD, Lodge B: Aneurysm of the splenic artery. *Gut* 1960; 1: 312-320.

[14] Dave SP, Reis ED, Hossain A, et al: Splenic artery aneurysm in the 1990s. *Ann Vasc Surg* 2000; 14:223-229.

[15] Pescarus R, Montreuil B, Bendavid Y: Giant splenic artery aneurysms: case report and review of the literature. *J Vasc Surg* 2005; 42:344-347.

[16] Lee PC, Rhee RY, et al. Management of splenic artery aneurysms: The significance of portal and essential hypertension. *J Am Cool Surg* 1999; 189: 483-490.

[17] Stanley JC, Wakefield TW, Graham LM, et al: Clinical importance and management of splanchnic artery aneurysms. *J Vasc Sur* 1986; 3:836-840.

[18] Sellke FW, Williams GB, Donovan DL, Clarke RE: Management of intra-abdominal aneurysms associated with periarteritis nodosa. *J Vasc Surg* 1986; 4:294-298.

[19] Ayalon A, Wiesner RH, Perkins JD, et al: Splenic artery aneurysms in liver transplant patients. *Transplantation* 1988; 45:386-389.

[20] Trastek VF, Pairolero PC, Joyce JW, et al: Splenic artery aneurysms. *Surgery* 1982; 91:694-699.

[21] Sadat U, Noor N, Tang T, Varty K: Emergency endovascular repair of ruptured visceral artery aneurysms. *World J Emerg Surg* 2007; 2:17.

[22] Hallett Jr JW: Splenic artery aneurysms. *Semin Vasc Surg* 1995; 8:321-326.

[23] Mattar SG, Lumsden AB: The management of splenic artery aneurysms: experience with 23 cases. *Am J Surg* 1995; 169:580-584.

[24] Alsheikhly A.S.: Ruptured True Aneurysm of the Splenic Artery: A Rare Cause of Haemoperitoneum: *The Middle East Journal of Trauma and Emergency medicine* 2008;8:197-199.

[25] Mattar SG, Lumsden AB: The management of splenic artery aneurysms: experience with 23 cases. *Am J Surg* 1995; 169:580-584.

[26] de Vries JE, Schattenkerk ME, Malt RA: Complications of splenic artery aneurysm other than intraperitonealrupture. *Surgery* 1982; 91:200-204.

[27] Wagner WH, Allins AD, Treiman RL, et al: Ruptured visceral artery aneurysms. *Ann Vasc Surg* 1997; 11:342-347.

[28] Trastek VF, Pairolero PC, Joyce JW, et al: Splenic artery aneurysm. *Surgery* 1982; 91:694-699.

[29] Barrett JM, Van Hooydonk JE, Boehm FH: Pregnancy-related rupture of arterial aneurysms. *Obstet Gynecol Surv* 1982; 37:557-566.

[30] Stanley JC, Fry WJ: Pathogenesis and clinical significance of splenic artery aneurysms. *Surgery* 1974; 76:898-909.

[31] Nosher JL, Chung J, Brevetti LS, et al: Visceral and renal artery aneurysms: a pictorial essay on endovascular therapy. *Radiographics* 2006; 26:1687-1704.

[32] Messina LM, Shanley CJ: Visceral artery aneurysms. *Surg Clin North Am* 1997; 77:425-442.

[33] Abbas MA, Stone WM, Fowl RJ, et al: Splenic artery aneurysms: two decades experience at Mayo Clinic. *Ann Vasc Surg* 2002; 16:442-449.

[34] Arca MJ, Gagner M, Heniford BT, et al: Splenic artery aneurysms: methods of laparoscopic repair. *J Vasc Surg* 1999; 30:184-188.

[35] Mastracci TM, Cadeddu M, Colopinto RF, Cina C: A minimally invasive approach to the treatment of aberrant splenic artery aneurysms: a report of two cases. *J Vasc Surg* 2005; 41:1053-1057.

[36] Huang IH, Zuckerman DA, Matthews JB: Occlusion of a giant splenic artery pseudoaneurysm with percutaneous thrombin-collagen injection. *J Vasc Surg* 2004; 40:574-577.

[37] Saltzberg SS, Maldonado TS, Lamparello PJ, et al: Is endovascular therapy the preferred treatment for all visceral artery aneurysms?. *Ann Vasc Surg* 2005; 19:507-515.

[38] Carroccio A, Jacobs TS, Faries P, et al: Endovascular treatment of visceral artery aneurysms. *Vasc Endovasc Surg* 2007; 41:373-382.

[39] LinkDP, Seibert JA, Gould J, Lantz BM. On-line monitoring of sequential blood flow reduction during splenic embolization. *Acta Radio* 1989; 30: 101–103.

[40] Tulsyan N, Kashyap VS, Greenberg RK, et al: The endovascular management of visceral artery aneurysms and pseudoaneurysms. *J Vasc Surg* 2007; 45:276-283.

[41] Sachdev U, Baril DT, Ellozy SH, et al: Management of aneurysms involving branches of the celiac and superior mesenteric arteries: a comparison of surgical and endovascular therapy. *J Vas Surg* 2006; 44:718-724.

[42] Pulli R, Dorigo W, Troisi N, et al: Surgical treatment of visceral artery aneurysms: a 25-year experience. *J Vasc Surg* 2008; 48:334-342.

[43] Gabelmann A, Gorich J, Merkle EM: Endovascular treatment of visceral artery aneurysms. *J Endovasc Ther* 2002; 9:38-47.

[44] Salam TA, Lumsden AB, Martin LG, Smith 3rd RB: Nonoperative management of visceral aneurysms and pseudoaneurysms. *Am J Surg* 1992; 164:215-219.

[45] Saltzberg SS, Maldonado TS, Lamparello PJ, et al: Is endovascular therapy the preferred treatment for all visceral artery aneurysms?. *Ann Vasc Surg* 2005; 19:507-515.

[46] Sachdev U, Baril DT, Ellozy SH, et al: Management of aneurysms involving branches of the celiac and superior mesenteric arteries: a comparison of surgical and endovascular therapy. *J Vasc Surg* 2006; 44:718-724.

[47] Szopinski P, Ciostek P, Pleban E, et al: Percutaneous thrombin injection to complete SMA pseudoaneurysm exclusion after failing of endograft placement. *Cardiovasc Intervent Radiol* 2005; 28:509-514.

[48] Carr SC, Pearce WH, Vogelzang RL, et al: Current management of visceral artery aneurysms. *Surgery* 1996; 120:627-633.
[49] Onohara T, Okadome K, Mii S, et al: Rupture of embolized coeliac artery pseudoaneurysm into the stomach: is coil embolization an effective treatment for coeliac anastomotic pseudoaneurysm?. *Eur J Vasc Surg* 1992; 6:330-332.

Chapter 9

Abdominal Aortic Aneurysms – Actual Therapeutic Strategies

Ionel Droc, Dieter Raithel and Blanca Calinescu

Additional information is available at the end of the chapter

1. Introduction

AAA is the thirteenth cause of death in UK accounting for 1.2% of male and 0.6 of female mortality, and the third cause of sudden death after coronary artery disease and stroke. [1-3]

Abdominal aortic aneurysms are identified in the elderly population; only a few patients die because of AAA rupture prior to the age of 60. The incidence of the disease in the general population is 60/1000 inhabitants [4] and between 1.8% and 6.6% in autopsies studies. In studies of natural history of AAA the rate of aneurysm rupture and death could exceed 60% within 3 years of the initial diagnosis. [5]

2. Pathogenesis

The pathogenesis of aortic aneurismal disease is multifactorial. There is no consensus as to the cause of aortic aneurysms. Hypertension exists in about half of patients and is obviously an aggravating condition. Tertiary syphilis was once an important cause of aneurysms, particularly of the ascending thoracic aorta, but is a less common cause now.

Genetic components have been identified in Marfan's syndrome and Ehlers Danlos disease. Even in the most common, degenerative, form of aortic aneurysms there is a genetic component. Familial clustering of aortic aneurysms is evident as up to 20% of patients have one or more first-degree relatives who have also suffered from the disease.[6] More studies are clearly needed to establish details of the genetic interplay in aortic aneurysms.

At times, an aneurysm may be caused by an extrinsic factor, such as an infection (micotic aneurysm) or trauma (pseudoaneurysm).

Traditional views states that most aneurysms were caused by degenerative atherosclerotic disease but it affects different layers of the aortic wall. Atherosclerosis mainly affects the intima, causing occlusive disease, while aortic aneurysm is a disease of the media and adventitia. They are distinct conditions that nonetheless often occur together.

Histologically, AAAs are characterized by chronic inflammation with destruction of the extracellular matrix, remodelling of the wall layers, and reduction in number of smooth muscle cells. The effectors of destruction are a group of enzymes capable of degrading the major connective tissue components: collagen, elastin, fibronectin, laminin and the proteoglycans.[7] The inflammatory infiltrate consists of macrophages as well as T and B lymphocytes, which excrete proteases and elastases causing wall degradation.[8] The reason for this migration is unclear.

Degradation of elastin has been associated with dilatation while rupture of the wall is related to collagen degradation. Experimental studies of elastase induced aneurysms indicate that an inflammatory reaction within the aortic media is crucial for aortic dilatation.

In both clinical and experimental studies, metalloproteinases (MMP), one of the most prominent group of elastases, have emerged as playing a role in the development of aortic aneurysms. [9,10] The MMPs are inhibited by the family of tissue inhibitors of metalloproteinases (TIMPs), including TIMP-1 and TIMP-2. An imbalance between the activated MMPs and their natural inhibitors may be responsible for the destruction of the aortic wall. Therapeutic trials with doxycycline, a MMP inhibitor, are ongoing and preliminary results are encouraging with less progression of aneurysmal size in treated patients.[11]

Commonly assessed in AAA are also proteins involved in, stimulated by or associated with thrombosis, for example, fibrinogen and D-dimer.[12]

A human biopsy study has confirmed the association between the extent of inflammation of the aortic wall and aortic diameter.[13] Interleukin-6 (IL-6), metalloproteinase-9 (MMP-9-gelatinase B) and C-reactive protein (CRP) are markers of inflammatory processes and have all been associated with AAA pathogenesis [13,14,15] as well as collagen type IV, fibronectin and other matrix proteins. High levels of MMP-9 and MMP-3 have been found in abdominal aortic aneurysmal tissue. Levels of MMP-9 are associated with aneurysmal size. [14,16,17] Hovsepian et al. Reported that MMP-9 plasma levels appeared to directly reflect the amount of MMP-9 produced within aneurysm tissue. MMP-9 plasma levels also decreased substantially after surgical AAA repair.[18]

Circulating concentrations of many kinds of biomarkers have been measured and compared in patients with abdominal aortic aneurysm (AAA) and subjects without AAA to assess their possible role in the pathogenesis or progression of AAA (Table 1). Circulating biomarkers could play a role in the diagnosis of AAA reflecting also the AAA activity in asymptomatic phases and may have a role in predicting subsequent progression and thus the prognosis of AAA.

Most investigated potential biomarkers show either no correlation or a weak correlation with the clinical course of AAA. Few have any potential for clinical use. Another limitation is related to the fact that many biomarkers for AAA are not disease specific; most of them also are markers for atherosclerosis.

Biomarker	Number of patients	Summary of findings	Author, year
MMP-9	36	Plasma MMP-9 may predict the natural history of AAA	Lindholt J. et al. 2000
MMP-9, MMP-2 TIMP-1, TIMP-2	76	Both MMP-2 and 9 failed to show relevance as serum markers for aortic dilatation.	Eugster T et al. 2005
	30 medium-sized ruptured AAA 30 large asymptomatic AAA (aAAA)	AAA rupture is associated with higher levels of MMP-9 in the aortic wall. There is no association to TIMP-1 or TIMP-2 levels. MMP-2 levels are positively, whereas MMP-9 levels are negatively correlated to aAAA. This may indicate that MMP-9 may have a determinant role in the AAA wall for the progression towards rupture, whereas MMP-2 pay a role for expansion.	E. Petersen et al. 2002 [19]
	37	Plasma levels of MMP-9 can accurately discriminate between patients with and without an endoleak with both high sensitivity and specificity. Anterior-postreior aneurysmal diameter (Dmax) was significantly larger in the endoleak group, however, plasma MMP-9 levels were not associated with Dmax or intraluminal thrombus volume.	F.A.M.V.I. Hellenthal et al.2012 [20]
MMP-9, MMP-1	52 non-ruptured AAA 16 ruptured AAA	The concentrations of MMP1 and MMP9 were significantly elevated in the plasma of ruptured AAA compared with non-ruptured AAA. There was no significant correlation between AAA diameter and enzyme concentration within the ruptured and non-ruptured cohorts.	W.R.W Wilson et al. 2008 [21]
P-Elastase	79	P-elastase was positively correlated with the mean annual AAA expansion rate.	Lindholt J. Et al. 2003
IFN-gamma	50	Elevated IFN-gamma concentrations seem to predict an increased rate of expansion in AAA.	Junoven J et al. 1997
TNF-alpha, IL-8	90	IL-8 and TNF-alpha can be used as endogenous markers of the process of AAA development.	Treska V et al. 2000
IL-6	7	In multivariate analysis the level of IL-6 was independently correlated with aortic diameter	Rodhe LE et al 1999
IL-6, MMP-9, CRP	213	No correlation was found between levels of circulating IL-6, MMP-9, CRP and the expansion of small-diameter AAAs, indicating no clinical use of these markers in AAA surveillance.	Karlsson L. Et al.2009 [22]

Biomarker	Number of patients	Summary of findings	Author, year
C-reactive Protein (CRP)	Sympt 52 Ruptured 62	No correlation. A significant elevation of CRP could be found in patients who presented symptoms or rupture of an AAA.	Domanivits H et al.2002
	545	CRP levels are elevated in larger aneurysms but do not appear to be associated with rapid expansion.	Norman P et al. 2004
	151	CRP did not correlate with size or expansion rate of AAA	Lindholt J et al 2001
Serum highly sensitive CRP	39	Serum hsCRP is associated with aneurysmal size.	Vainas T et al. 2003
CRP, alpha 1-antitripsin	35 AAA patients 35 controls	A positive correlation was found between CRP and AAA diameter and alpha 1-antitripsin and AAA growth. Alpha 1-antitripsin may be a promising biomarker of AAA growth.	M. Vega de Ceniga et al.2009 [23]
D-dimer, fibrinogen/fibrin	36	The largest diameter of AAA is correlated with the preoperative levels of D-dimer and FDP	Yamazuni K et al.1998
	834 cases with AAA and 6971 controls for fibrinogen 264 cases with AAA and 403 controls for D-dimer.	Plasma fibrinogen and D-dimer concentrations are likely to be higher in cases with AAA than control subjects. Higher plasma fibrinogen and D-dimer concentrations may be associated with the presence of AAA.	Takagi H. Et al. 2009 [12]
	110 patients with AAA 110- controls	Fibrinogen was positively correlated with AAA size (r =0.323; p<0.01) and the percentage of intra-luminal thrombus occupying the lumen (r =0.358; p<0.05).	Al-Barjas et al. 2006 [24]
Insulin-like Growth Factor 1 (IGF-I)	115 small AAAs	Serum IGF-I, but not IGF-II, correlated positively with AAA size and AAA growth. IGF-I levels may serve as a novel biomarker for the natural history of AAA.	J.S. Lindholt et al. 2011 [25]

Table 1. Summary of published studies reporting the role of circulating biomarkers in the growth and rupture of AAA

Active investigations continue to identify markers other than size that would predict a risk of rupture. Circulating biomarkers could also indicate optimal intervals between the surveillance intervals. Finally, the identification of biomarkers also may identify potential pathogenic pathways, and thus may open possibilities for pharmacological inhibition of growth, and provide a tool for monitoring this inhibition.[26]

In the future, extended longitudinal studies will be necessary to assess the true potential of matrix-turnover and other biomarkers. New methods, including proteomics and genome wide association studies, may identify new pathways and new potential biomarkers.

3. Treatment

Surgical repair was first reported in 1962 and still remains the treatment with the best long-term results. The surgical technique is illustrated in **Figure 1**. It is a major surgical procedure done under general anaesthesia, usually consisting of a midline laparotomy and cross clamping of the aorta and iliac vessels.

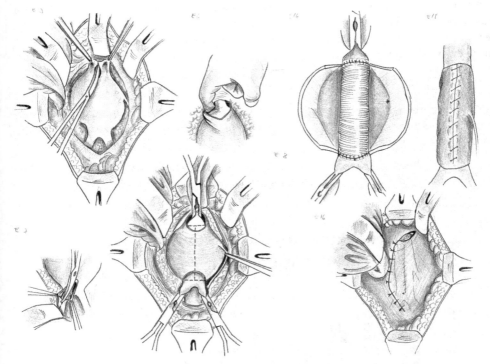

Figure 1. Open surgery technique for AAA

The mortality of elective surgery is between 3 and 7%. These rates increase significantly in patients with comorbidities, particularly with coronary artery disease and carotid artery disease. Surgical results are impaired by chronic renal failure and COPD.

Increasing age is an important adverse determinant of mortality in both ruptured and intact aneurysms.

In the USA statistics indicate that more than 15000 deaths/year are caused by aneurysm rupture.

This is the reason why there are screening studies among the target population in order to save lives and decrease health costs. The great interest is to detect and treat the AAA before rupture but the problem is that most of them are asymptomatic.

Because open surgery has non-negligible mortality and postoperative complications associated with a long hospital stay (10.8 days average) scientists tried to develop alternative methods to treat this disease addressing those cases with surgical high risk.

Minimally invasive techniques were developed in order to exclude the aneurysm from the circulation and to provide a new circulator channel towards the legs. Potential applications of endovascular grafts have been found in all areas of vascular surgery but their use for aortic aneurysms was the first to be explored. Endovascular aneurysm repair (EVAR) is an alternative to open surgery in the management of AAA. Juan Parodi and colleagues performed the first endovascular aneurysm repair in Argentina in 1991 [27,28]. Two decades after, the technique has evolved immensely and new devices developed allowing to a greater number of patients to be treated with EVAR. Repair of aortic abdominal aneurysm (AAA) is performed to prevent progressive expansion and rupture. [27, 29 30]

EVAR is progressively replacing open surgery and now accounts for more than half AAA repairs [31] as for example endovascular repair of AAA in Kaiser Hawaii Hospital (USA) was 50% in 2004 of the surgical activity.

A study published in November 2011 identifies the rate of endovascular treatment for AAA in different countries during 2005-2009 (**Figure 2**), whose prospective data were included in

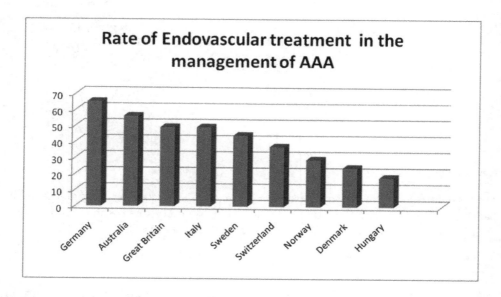

Figure 2. Rate of EVAR in the management of AAA in different countries

the VASCUNET database [32]. The study shows a rapid and extensive implementation of the endovascular treatment, with the advent of studies with favourable results in this direction.

EVAR in addition to the advantage of being a minimally invasive method and as such preferred by the patients, has many proven benefits compared with traditional open surgery: low rate of peri- and postoperative mortality and morbidity, shorter hospital stay, significantly reduced intraoperative blood loss and faster recovery. [33, 34, 35] One drawback is the significantly higher reintervention rate compared to open repair.

4. Evidence base for EVAR

In order to evaluate this new method there are registries [36] (retrospective studies) as: RETA (registry of endovascular treatment for aneurysms) in the UK, started in 1996 [37], EUROSTAR also started in 1996 [38], the Lifeline registry in the USA started in 1998 [39]. There are also randomized, controlled, multicenter trials: EVAR 1 and 2 initiated in 1999 and DREAM (Dutch randomized endovascular aneurysm management) started in 2000.

In RETA, 31 UK centers submitted data. From January 1996 to December 1998 611 cases were enrolled. Four percent received an aortic tube device, 60% an aorto-iliac device and 36% an aorto uni-iliac device with femoro-femoral crossover graft. The objectives were to assess early morbidity and mortality. Conversion to open repair was in 5% of cases. The overall mortality was 7% vs. 12% for open surgery. Endoleaks were more common in larger aneurysms (2% if aneurysm diameter was < 6 cm and 10% if it was > 6 cm) [37].

EUROSTAR (European collaboration on stent graft techniques for aortic aneurysm repair) Registry was established in 1996. The results were published in JVS in October 2000, 88 European centers have contributed, enrolling 2464 patients with a main follow up of 12.19 months. The 30 days mortality was 3.1%. The cumulative risk of late conversion was 2.1%/year and of rupture 1%/year. The significant factors for rupture were: type I endoleak, type III endoleak, graft migration and postoperative kinking of the endograft. The feasibility rate of the procedure was 97% of patients using first and second generation devices. The rate of late failure of the devices was 3%/year.[38,40]

The Lifeline registry was established in 1998 in the USA and the results were published in JVS in July 2005. The end point was to evaluate the long-term outcome of patients treated with EVAR using 5 devices who had FDA approval (Guidant Ancure, Medtronic AneuRx, Gore Excluder, Endologix PowerLink, Cook Zenith). It enrolled 2664 patients with EVAR vs. 334 open repair control patients. The 30 day mortality of EVAR was 1.7% which was not different from surgical control (1.4%), this in spite of the EVAR patients who were significantly older and sicker (more comorbidities). The risk of rupture of the aneurysm after EVAR was 3 times higher (2.1%) in women than in men (0.7%). The risk of rupture of the AAA remained stable over a 6 year period at a level of 1%/year. The surgical conversion rate was 3% at a year and 5% at 6 years (low). All this shows that EVAR is safe and effective in preventing aneurysm rupture and avoiding AAA related death. [39]

The most known and discussed randomized, controlled, multicentre trials are the UK EVAR1 and 2 which were initiated in 1999 and published in "The Lancet" in 2004 [41] and 2005 [42]. EVAR 1 compares endovascular procedures vs. open repair. A great number of patients (2068) were enrolled, aged over 60 years with a non ruptured AAA and who had an aneurysm of more than 5.5 cm in CT scan diameter. Morphological suitability for EVAR [43] and choice of the stent graft was decided by each center (41 centers enrolled). The 30-day mortality rate was 1.7% compared with 4.7% for open surgery. The secondary interventions were 9.8 for EVAR and 5.8 for open repair. Patients unfit for open repair because of significant comorbidities were randomized for EVAR or best medical treatment in the EVAR 2 trial. 338 patients aged 60 years or older with an AAA >5.5 cm in diameter were enrolled. The primary end point was aneurysm related mortality, postoperative complications and hospital costs. The risk of rupture is 25%/year for aneurysms with diameters greater than 6 cm. The 30-day mortality was 9% in EVAR group and in the non intervention group was 9.0 / 100 pers / year. There was no significant difference between the EVAR group and non intervention group for all cause mortality.

The DREAM trial initiated in 2000 enrolled 345 patients considered suitable for both types of treatment. The 30-day mortality after EVAR was 1.2% compared with 4.6% for open surgery. The results were published in 2002 in Journal of Cardiovascular Surgery [44, 45].

The Veteran open vs. endovascular repair (OVER) trial started enrollment in October 2002 in the US. It was design to enroll 5 years followed by a 4 year follow up. In total a 9 years survey. The primary outcome is long-term survival and secondary outcomes included morbidity, procedure failures and need for secondary procedures and costs. 33 centers are participating, 684 patients were enrolled in September 2006 and the investigators expect 900 by the end of the study. Patients enrolled had aneurysms of more than 5cm and were candidates for both procedural types. [46]

The French trial *"Anevrisme Chirurgie vs Endoprothese"* (ACE) also had the same enrollment conditions and primary and secondary end points.

In OVER and ACE trials were used newer devices for treating AAA than those used in EVAR 1 and DREAM (procedures performed between 1999-2003)[46]. The Gore Excluder and Medtronic AneuRx represent 2/3 from the devices used in OVER compared with only 11% used in EVAR 1.

Speaking about costs the shorter ITU and hospital stay in the EVAR group, with initial comparable costs, the cost per patient over 4 years is higher in EVAR because the cost of the endograft and subsequent of secondary interventions **(Figure 3)**[43].

In summary, EVAR has lower perioperative mortality but there is no difference in long term overall mortality. This procedure is associated with 10% risk of aneurysm related complications/ year, but they can be solved by further endovascular reinterventions [43].

EVAR is a safe, effective and durable treatment for infrarenal aortic aneurysms with suitable anatomy.

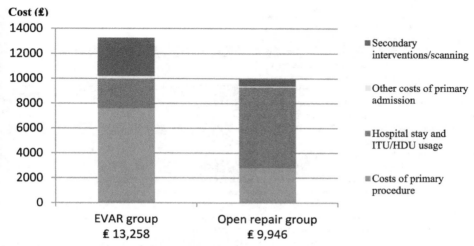

Figure 3. EVAR costs per patient (modified after [43])

5. Indications and anatomical suitability

Patient selection is an important element of successful EVAR. We should carefully investigate and consider the anatomy of the abdominal aorta, the relationship with the emergence of the renal arteries, the calibre, tortuosity and calcifications of the iliac arteries. The misevaluation of morphological aspects can lead to immediate or late failure of the procedure. With the refinement of medical devices (multislice CT scan with 3D reconstruction, substraction angiography, sophisticated computer data analysis), we can detect all the morphological modifications in the aneurismal area in segments immediately adjacent.

The Clinical Practice Guidelines of the European Society for Vascular Surgery on the management of AAA, published in April 2011, sets out a series of recommendations in all aspects of diagnosis and management strategies of AAA (Figure 4,5) [47].

There is a consensus that in the case of small aneurysms, with a diameter between 3.0-3.9 cm, the risk of rupture in negligible. Therefore, these aneurysms do not require surgery, supervision by Doppler Ultrasound at regular intervals being sufficient. The management of the AAA with a diameter between 4.0 – 5.5 was determined by two multicenter, randomised, controlled studies, that compared the natural evolution of these aneurysms versus early intervention: UK Small Aneurysm Trial (UKSAT) and American Aneurysm Detection and Management Study (ADAM) respectively [48, 49] and a smaller study, that compared endovascular treatment versus surveillance, the CAESAR study [50]. The PIVOTAL study including aneurysms with diameters between 4.0- 5.0 cm compared the endovascular treatment versus Doppler Ultrasound surveillance [51].

Medium-term results of these studies did not indicate a statistically significant difference in terms of overall mortality at 5 years, the results being similar in the long-term, at 12 years

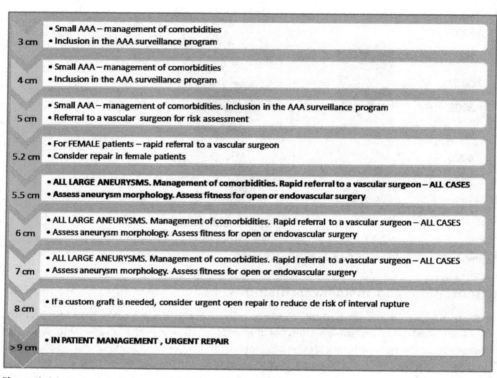

Figure 4. Management strategy of AAA according to the size of the aneurysm (modified after [47])

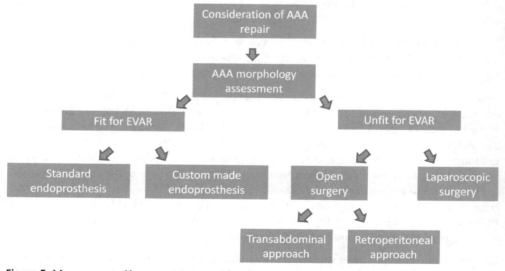

Figure 5. Management of large aneurysms, with a diameter ≥5,5 cm (modified after [47])

[48, 52]. The rupture rate of the aneurysms was 1% in the surveillance group and the overall mortality rate was 5,6% in the early intervention group.

The results of the above mentioned large studies, UKSAT and ADAM were recently included in the COCHRANE study, that underlines the safety and through this the benefits of the Doppler ultrasound surveillance of the AAA with a diameter between 4.0 and 5.5 cm [53].

Performing Doppler Ultrasound surveillance of small aneurysms (4.0-5.5 cm) is safe and recommended for asymptomatic aneurysms. If the aneurysm reaches the 5.5 cm diameter limit, measured by Doppler ultrasound (in male patients), it becomes symptomatic or there is an annual diameter increase of >1cm/year, the patient must be immediately referred for further investigation to the specialised vascular surgery department.

As highlighted, the diameter of the AAA establishes the moment for intervention, but this criteria alone is not enough to establish the indication for the endovascular treatment of the AAA. With new treatment methods new complications occur, requiring further investigations in order to assess the feasibility of the AAA for EVAR. The morphological criteria of the AAA are the ones that can establish or exclude the indication of EVAR. The failure to comply with these criteria, requested also in the instruction manuals of the endoprostheses currently on the market may lead to the increase of the peri- and postoperative complication, reintervention and post-EVAR mortality rate.

An average 34% of AAA is not eligible for EVAR, most of them because of an adverse morphology. [54]

The universal classification system defines the aneurysm in relation with the origin of renal arteries:

- infrarenal, with a segment of normal (undilated) aorta named neck
- pararenal or juxtarenal, when aneurysm originate just after the renals
- suprarenal, the aneurysm includes the origin of renals or above without involvement of the superior mesenteric artery

Another classification employed for EUROSTAR and DREAM trials is shown in **figure 6,** taking into account the distance from the renals and the bifurcation of the aorta as well as the involvement of iliac arteries (the common iliac artery, arriving or not to the bifurcation of iliac arteries, occlusion or stenosis of the common iliac arteries).

The French system proposed by Kieffer & Chiche (2005) is also based on the distal extension of the aneurysm and is comparable with the EUROSTAR classification (Type I-V).

The proximal neck is by far one of the most important anatomic finding in planning an endovascular procedure. It can be classified as shown in **figure 7.**

The diameter of the neck, its length, shape and angulation are to be considered. Aortic neck angulation is defined as the angle between the axes of the proximal infrarenal aorta and the longitudinal axis of the aneurysm. It is classified as: mild < 40 degrees, moderate < 60dgr, and severe > 60dgr.

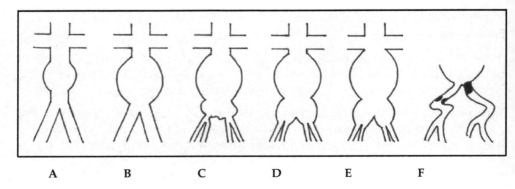

Figure 6. Classification of AAA (modified after [40])

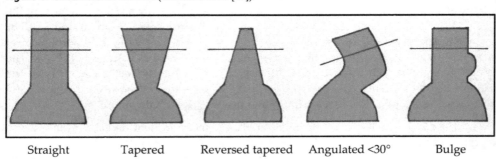

Straight   Tapered   Reversed tapered   Angulated <30°   Bulge

Figure 7. Morphology of the aortic neck (modified after [40])

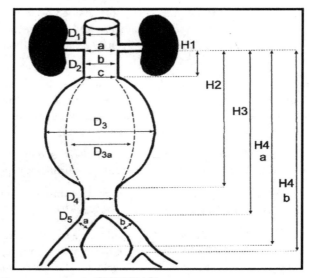

Figure 8. Preoperative measurements (EUROSTAR)

The neck is the place where the endoprotheses are fixed and sealed. Seal is the apposition of the outer surface of the endograft to the luminal surface of the aorta in order to exclude the aneurysm sac from the systemic pressure. Fixation is the counterforce that prevents migration and helps to maintain seal.

Concerning the iliac arteries, the landing zone of the majority of grafts, we are interested in patency and diameter, length of the common iliac artery, shape or aneurismal, angulation or tortuosity and calcifications.

Figure 8 shows a preoperative scheme for planning an endovascular repair showing all the anatomical features discussed above.(after [40])

5. Types of endoprostheses in use

The grafts are classified in different manners. From the anatomic point of view, they can be: bifurcated (Ao bi-iliac), Ao – uni-iliac and tube (for Ao – Aortic – these were the most used, but now they are out of the market). They can be modular (most of them) or unibody (Powerlink).

Figure 9 shows the images of some endoprosthesis in use today: modular (a,b,c) and unibody (d).

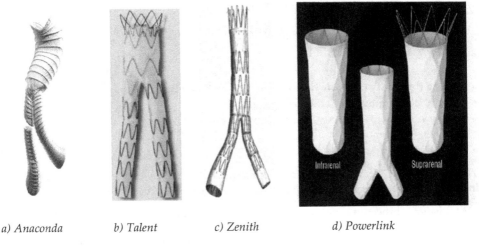

a) Anaconda   *b) Talent*   *c) Zenith*   *d) Powerlink*

Figure 9. Most used endoprosthesis

The modular devices have at least two component grafts. The main body deployed on the neck of the aneurysm *("hanging from the Aorta")* and the two legs that arrives on the common iliac arteries. The unibody prostheses build up the endoluminal channel from the bottom to the top, sitting on the aortic bifurcation (concept of anatomical fixation) [55]. This prevents distal migration of the endoprostheses.

The characteristics of the most used endografts [56, 57] are shown in the **table 2:**

Endograft characteristics							
Device	Material	Configuration	Deployment	Fixation	Aortic graft diam.	Iliac graft diam.	Supra-renal stent
Zenith (Cook)	Polyester	Modular	Self-expanding	Compression-fit and barbs	22-36	8-24	Yes
Talent (Medtronic)	Polyester	Modular	Self-expanding	Compression-fit	24-34	8-24	Yes
Excluder (Gore)	ePTFE	Modular	Self-expanding	Compression-fit and anchors	23/26/28.5	12-14.5	No
Anaconda (Terumo)	Twilleave	Modular	Self-expanding	Compression-fit and hooks	19.5-34	9-18	No
Powerlink (Endologix)	ePTFE	One-piece	Self-expanding	Compression-fit	25/28	16	Optional
E-Vita (Jotec)	Polyester	Modular	Self-expanding	Compression-fit	24/34	14-26	yes

Table 2. The characteristics of the most used endografts [56, 57]

The characteristics of an ideal stent graft are:

- Low overall cost,
- Stent-graft size ranging,
- Long durability (metallic ultrastructure + graft material),
- Good biocompatibility and sealing capacity,
- Delivery device flexibility, lowest delivery device size,
- Radial force stability,
- Customization

The new results of the endovascular management of AAA (by type of endograft) are shown in **table 3** (retrospective or prospective studies) published in 2010 [58-63].

EVAR is not a procedure without complications[64-66]. One of the most redoubtable are the *endoleak* [67]. They are defined as persistence of the blood flow outside the lumen of the endograft, but within the aneurismal sac [68]. An endoleak may perfuse the aneurysm sac leading to aneurysm expansion and may be rupture. It represents the inability to obtain or maintain secure seal between the aortic wall and the graft [1]. The incidence of endoleaks is in range of 14%. They are classified in four types (from I to IV) [see the **table 4** [1] modified].

The technique of introduction and deployment of the endograft is shown in **figure 10**. The access sites are the two femoral arteries. The anaesthesia required is general anaesthesia or loco-regional (peridural) [69].

Device	Author	Study Type	No cases	Period	Outcome		
					Peri OP mortality	Limb patency 24months	Clinical success
Anaconda (Terumo)	Freyrie [58]	Prospective single center	127	2005-2009	0	96,7	100
Excluder (Gore)	Ghotbi [59]	Retro-spective	100	2006-2009	0	100	100
Endourant (Medtronic)	Bockler [60]	"Engage" prospective	180	2008-2009	1,7	100	99,4
Zenith (Cook)	Bequemin [61]	Prospective single center	212	2000-2004	0,9		99,5
Powerlink (Endologix)	Krajcer [62]	Prospective single center	50	2008-2010	0	100	98
Evita (Jotec)	Moula-kakis [63]	Retro-spective single center	30	2008-2009	0	100	100

Table 3.

I. Attachment site leaks
- Proximal end of endograft
- Distal end of endograft
- Iliac occlude [plug]
II. Branch leaks (collateral back bleeding)
- simple (one)
- complex (two or more branches)
III. Graft defect (modular dissociation)
- minor < 2mm
- major ≥ 2 mm
IV. Graft material porosity

Table 4. Classification of Endoleaks [1]

Both types I and III are significant risk factors for late aneurysm rupture and should be treated. Types II are considered benign and type IV usually resolves spontaneously during the post procedure period.

With this procedure, we can reduce blood lost (using also devices like the cell-saver) and consequent transfusion requirement, ITU and hospital stay. More patients can be treated where comorbidity previously excluded them. The follow-up is done by using CT scan exams at 1, 3, 6 and 12 months after the procedure. There are changes in the aneurysm volume after endovascular repair in terms of shrinking [61,70,71].

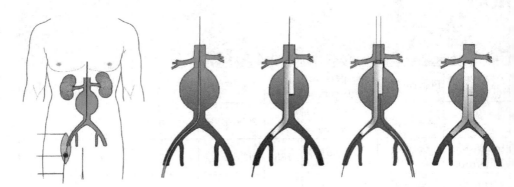

Figure 10. Schema of modular endograft deployment

6. Operative data and results (Nürnberg experience and Army's Clinic Center for Cardiovascular Diseases, Bucharest)

We have conducted a prospective, randomized study starting from 1994, including patients diagnosed with infrarenal aortic aneurysm with a diameter ≥ 5.5 cm. The purpose of this study was to assess the results of abdominal aortic aneurysm repair of two large volume centers, in terms of perioperative, early and midterm complications, reintervention rate and mortality.

Exclusion criteria were: Presence of comorbidities that could affect the postoperative surveillance: Renal insufficiency with serum creatinine level > 1.5 mg/dl, serum urea > 50 mg/dl, mental illnesses, hypersensitivity to the contrast agent, unable to be followed as an outpatient, claustrophobia, the presence of previously implanted metal devices: pace makers, mechanical heart valves etc.

Collected data: The collected data was entered in an excel database. Patient demographics and other variables were introduced, like:

- Qualitative variables: endovascular treatment indication, name and type of prosthesis used, vascular access method (percutaneous puncture of the femoral artery, surgical incision, temporary iliac conduit), type of anaesthesia, postoperative complications occurred (endoleak, endograft migration, kinking)
- Continuous quantitative variables: pre- and postoperative data on aneurysm morphology determined by CTA preoperatively and by DUS and CTA postoperatively (maximal anterior-posterior and transverse dimension of the aneurysm sac, length of the aneurysm, size and morphological changes of the aneurysm neck, the distance between the aneurysm and the emergence of the renal arteries, common iliac artery length and diameter) duration of intervention, the amount of blood loss, reinterventions.

In Nürnberg, we started endovascular treatment in 1994 with Ancure stent-graft. In our 14–years experience of 1502 cases (ending dec. 2007) we have used 13 different endografts.

From them, 1391 were men and 111 women, with a mean age of 71.5 years (41-98). The median follow up was 41 months (1.0-98) and the AAA had a mean diameter of 52.4 cm. For short and angulated necks we prefer now the Powerlink (Irvine, CA, USA) device, which we have started in 1999 [72]. Ending Dec. 2007, 519 cases were done using Powerlink grafts.

The 30 day mortality was 1.7%. The total reintervention rate was 5.3%, while no distal migration, conversion or post Evar rupture occurred. Using this device we arrive to treat endovascularly 85-90% of the infrarenal AAAs in our hospital.

At the **Army's Clinic Center for Cardiovascular Diseases,** Bucharest, between July 2008 - December 2010, 17 patients underwent EVAR for Abdominal Aortic Aneurysm (AAA), with age range between 49-82 years and aneurysm mean diameter 7.1 ± 0,5 cm (range: 5.4 – 8.2 cm) [73].

The preoperative assessment was achieved using Doppler Ultrasound (DUS), Multislice CT, and sometimes DSA (Digital Substraction Angiography). The measurements for the graft type and dimensions were done according to the Multislice CT analyzing. (**Figure 11 a, b and c**).

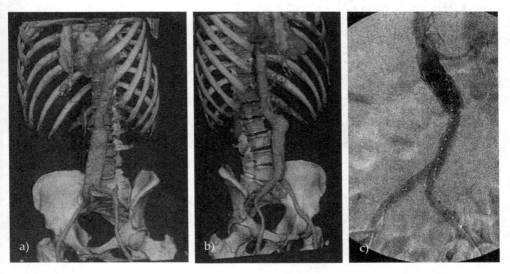

Figure 11. a), b) Preoperative multislice CT of a infrarenal AAA, with a suitable anatomy (2.2 cm neck length, no involvement of iliac arteries, 5.3 cm transversal diameter. **c)** Preoperative substraction angiography – with a catheter measuring the real length of the Aorta

The EVAR devices used for these patients were:

- Anaconda (Vascutek, Terumo, Inchinnan, Scotland)-1 patient
- Talent (Medtronic, Santa Rosa, CA, USA) -3 patients
- Powerlink (Endologix, Irvine,CA, USA) – 7 patients
- EVITA (Iotec, Hechingen, Germany)- 6 patients.

The access was bifemoral, through open femoral incision, with peridural anaesthesia.

Until present they followed our institutions surveillance protocol, that consisted of both DUS and CTA examination at 1,3,6,12 months and yearly after EVAR. None of them went through all of the surveillance dates (due to high examination costs) but each has at least 3 sets of examinations, one set consisting of both DUS and CTA.

The technical success rate was 100%, with no perioperative and postoperative complications regarding endoleaks, graft migration and graft component failure. 4 patients had access site complications, 3 had groin haematomas that reabsorbed after approximately 1 week and 1 returned with an infection at the level of the inguinal incision, which resolved also with wound care. There were no conversions to open repair up to present. The stent-graft patency rate at this point at these patients is 100%.

Figures 12 and **13** show two cases of AAAs treated with two different devices and two different strategies: Anaconda (Terumo) device and Powerlink (Endologix) stent graft.

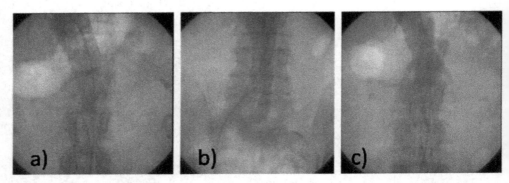

Figure 12. AAA treated with Powerlink Endograft **a)** Proximal extension; **b)** Main body of the stent-graft; **c)** The two iliac segments of Powerlink® system

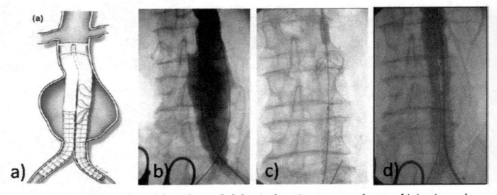

Figure 13. a) Anaconda endograft for infrarenal abdominal aortic aneurysm therapy; **b)** Angiography at the beginning of the procedure; **c)** The main body of the stent; **d)** The two iliac Anaconda system

7. Particular situations

7.1. Ruptured AAA

In open repair of ruptured AAAs the perioperative mortality ranges between 30% and 65%[74,75].Emergency EVAR is an alternative in selected patients with RAAA. The first report of emergency repair of an AAA was in 1994. Possible advantages are avoiding general anesthesia and laparotomy. Though a major inconvenient is the need of an endovascular team to be available at all times and to assess the preoperative CT scan in order to choose the size of the device. Following the emergent CT scan the anatomical suitability for EVAR was evaluated, including the access vessels [76].Several modular or unibody devices can be used but aorto-uni-iliac devices with subsequent fem-fem crossover bypass and occlusion of contralateral iliac artery could also be used. Veith [77] reported in 2009 a series of 57 patients with R-AAA treated endovascularly. 25 of these patients received the **VI graft** (distributed in Europe by Datascope-Maquet), made of a large Palmaz stent attached to a PTFE graft. This graft is used in aortofemoral configuration. This graft is "a one size fits most "because the proximal diameter can vary from 20 to27mm depending on the balloon inflation pressure. The periprocedural mortality was only 12,3%,inspite of serious medical comorbidities of the patients.

In the series reported by Kapma in 2005 on 253 patients treated with E-EVAR vs open surgery the perioperative mortality was lower (13%) in the Evar group compared with OR (30% p=0,021).According to the SVS practical guidelines [31] E-EVAR should be considered for treatment of a R-AAA, if anatomically feasible, with a **strong** level of recommendation and a **moderate** quality of evidence.

7.2. Juxtarenal AAA

Juxtarenal AAA have short (11-15mm), or very short (< 10mm) necks. The anatomically unsuitable AAAs has short and/or angulated necks. They have a high risk of stent graft distal migration and proximal type I endoleak, because the inability to provide a sufficient proximal landing zone to secure fixation and seal. The strategy for treating this challenging AAAs is to build up the endoluminal exclusion system from the aortic bifurcation to the renal artery level with suprarenal fixation. At Nürnberg Hospital we used the Powerlink unibody bifurcated stent graft with a long suprarenal cuff. A Palmaz stent can be used for proximal fixation in hostile necks (short necks with severe angulation).

Suprarenal fixation does not lead to a significant increase of acute renal events (renal insufficiency, high blood pressure) compared with infrarenal fixation [72]

Figure 14 shows an angiography of AAA treated with a Powerlink graft with suprarenal fixation; for better sealing a proximal ballooning at the end of the procedure was performed.

7.3. AAA with iliac extension

The iliac extension of the AAAs can put technical problems in choosing the graft, especially if the iliac aneurysm reaches the bifurcation of the iliac artery (fig.11a). In this situation, the

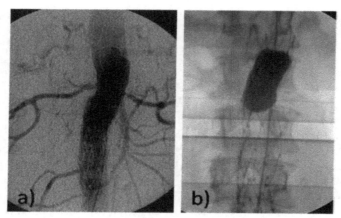

Figure 14. a) After suprarenal prox. Cuff; **b)** Proximal balloning. Fenestrated grafts are now available to treat juxtarenal AAA [78-80]

leg of the graft should land on the external iliac artery, covering the hypogastric artery (post-operation complications can occur like buttock claudication). In the case of planning to cover one hypogastric artery, we should close the artery (by coiling for ex.) a few days before implanting the endograft, in order to prevent distal type II endoleak.

Figure 15 shows a 72 year old patient treated at the Army's Center for Cardiovascular Diseases, using a Powerlink graft with left iliac graft extension - left hypogastric artery was occluded with coils 24h before the intervention.

In order to preserve the hypogastric artery, custom made, fenestrated or branched endografts can be used. Although this procedure was performed to prevent pelvic ischemia, this is not always the case. **Figure 16** presents a case of a 75 year old male patient with AAA

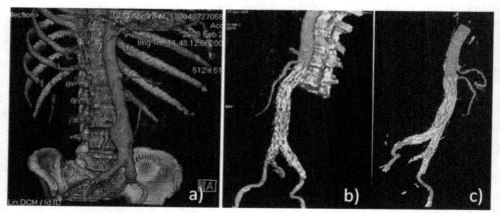

Figure 15. Patient O.P., 72 years old, preoperative multislice CT; **a)** AAA with left iliac extension; **b)** multislice CT-Scan at 3 months after EVAR with PowerLink endoprosthesis; **c)** multislice CT-Scan 2 years after EVAR with PowerLink endoprosthesis.

treated by EVAR with a fenestrated endograft that presented to our department with buttock claudication 6 months after EVAR. The performed angiography evidentiated an occluded right hypogastric artery. Conservative treatment with Vasaprostan 20µg was instituted with good results.

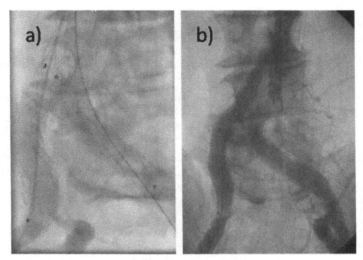

Figure 16. 75 year old male patient with AAA treated by EVAR Completion angiography after EVAR using a fenestrated endograft for the right hypogastric artery. **b)** Angiography performed 6 months after the intervention showing an occluded right hypogastric artery.

7.4. AAA and comorbidities: Coronary artery disease, carotid stenosis.

It is well known today that cardiac complications of patients with AAAs treated endovascularly is between 3 to 7%[31]. In order to avoid useless coronarographic investigations , we have to identify clinical parameters to indicate prior myocardial revascularization (surgery or stenting). Kieffer and Coriat, in a study published in 1999, on 270 patients operated for terminal Aorta pathology (aneurismal or stenotic) show an incidence of 55% of coronary stenosis in the AAA population which requires in 25% of cases myocardial revascularization. The risk factors which were identified were age >65 years and history of myocardial infarction. Stable angina with left main disease, or triple-vessel disease, as well as patients with two vessel disease that includes proximal LAD are candidates for preoperative coronary revascularization. The coronary intervention should be done prior to AAA treatment in one month interval. However the perioperative mortality can arrive to 25% (with extracorporeal circulation and cardiac arrest)

The carotid stenosis with a hemodynamic impact has a prevalence of 10.5%in the AAA patients.

Coronary and/or carotid lesions, treated or not, represent a significant risk factor for postoperative death. For this, systematic preoperative screening is mandatory [81,82].

Steinmetz published in 2008 an analysis of outcome after using high risk criteria selection to surgery vs. EVAR [83].The conclusion was that high risk criteria cannot be decisive in the choice of treatment.

8. Future developments

8.1. Totally percutaneous procedures

Because local groin wound complications as a result of the exposure of the two common femoral arteries are not negligible [84], surgeons and engineers tried to develop alternative access techniques. One of them is the fully percutaneous procedure. The main device available is Perclose ProstarXL(Abbott). For technical success patient and device selection should be done. Severe femoral artery calcification, scarred groins, femoral artery aneurysms are contraindications for the use of these devices. The overall related complications were 4.4%. Among them infection and artery trombose are the most redoubtable. The hospital stay is shorter in patients undergoing P-EVAR (2.7 days vs. 3.5 days) compared with EVAR. In conclusion, P-EVAR appears safe and effective in selected patients.

8.2. MRI devices

A new research field in our days is based on the hypotheses that the endografts can be visualized and navigated in vivo solely under Rt-MRI(real time magnetic resonance imaging). MRI can provide immediate assessment of endograft apposition and aneurysm exclusion. MRI offers also better soft tissue visualization, detecting type I endoleaks by depiction of complex 3D anatomy.

The technique is now applicable on murine models of AAA [85]. They have used a passive commercial endograft, image based on metal MRI artefacts, and active homemade endografts incorporating MRI receiver coils (antennae). Active devices proved to be most useful. The MRI images proved graft apposition and aneurysm exclusion. MRI imaging also permits immediate post-procedural anatomical and functional evaluation of the successful procedure.

In conclusion, MRI may be equivalent or superior to computed tomography for procedure planning and surveillance of the endografts. Future development of active devices is required, in order to have a commercial graft that can be used in clinical testing and practice.

9. Conclusions

Our results show that in the modern era of abdominal aortic aneurysm treatment EVAR is an appropriate treatment for selected patients, especially those at high risk for open surgical repair.

The future of EVAR as the potential gold standard for aortic aneurysm therapy rests upon the vision and creativity of both surgeons and technology innovators to realize the potential of endovascular interventions, and take them toward a broader and more effective portfolio of techniques and devices that will define the XXI-st Century Endovascular Aortic Surgery.

Author details

Ionel Droc* and Blanca Calinescu
Cardiovascular Surgery Department, Army's Clinic Center for Cardiovascular Diseases, Bucharest, Romania

Dieter Raithel
Klinikum Nürnberg Sud, Nürnberg, Germany

10. References

[1] Jaunoo S (2008) Endovascular aneurysm repair (EVAR). International Journal of Surgery. 6:266-269.

[2] Wyatt M.G (1999) Aneurysmal disease. In: Davies A.H, editor. Vascular Surgery Highlights 1998-1999. Oxford: Health Press. pp. 41-48.

[3] Garcia-Madric C, Josa M, Riambau V, Mestres C.A, Muntana J, Mulet J (2004) Endovascular versus open surgical repair of abdominal aortic aneurysm: a comparison of early and intermediate results in patients suitable for both techniques. Eur J Vasc Endovasc Surg. 28:365-372.

[4] Melton L, Bickerstaff L, Hollier L et al. (1984) Changing incidence of abdominal aortic aneurysms: A population-based study. Am J Epidemiol. 120:379-386.

[5] Reilly J.M, Tilson M.D (1989) Incidence and etiology of abdominal aortic aneurysms. Surg Clin North Am. 69:705-711.

[6] Pannu H, Fadulu V.T, Chang J et al. (2005) Mutations in transforming growth factor-beta receptor type II cause familial thoracic aortic aneurysms and dissections. Circulation.112:513-520.

[7] Busuttil R.W, Rinderbriecht H, Flesher A et al. (1982) Elastase activity: the role of elastase in aortic aneurysm formation. J Surg Res. 32:214-217.

[8] Safi H.J (2007) Thoracic aortic aneurysms: classification, incidence, etiology, natrural history and results. In: Lumsden A.B, Lin P.H, Changyi Chen, Parodi J.C, editors. Advanced Endovascular Therapy of Aortic Disease. Malden: Blackwell Publishing. pp. 25-30

[9] Ailawadi G, Eliason J.L, Upchurch G.R Jr. (2003) Current concepts in the pathogenesis of abdominal aortic aneurysm. J.Vasc Surg. 38:584-588.

[10] Grootenboer N, Bosch J.L, Hendriks J.M, van Sambeek M.R.H.M (2009) Epidemiology, Aetiology, Risk of Rupture and Treatment of Abdominal Aortic Aneurysms: Does Sex Matter?. Eur J Vasc Endovasc Surg. 38:278-284.

[11] Mosorin M, Junoven J, Biancari F, Satta J, Surcel H.M, Leinonen M et al. (2001) Use of doxycycline to decrease the growth rate of abdominal aortic aneurysms: A randomized, double-blind, placebo-controlled pilot study. J Vasc Surg. 34:606-610.

[12] Takagi H, Manabe H, Kawai N, Goto S, Umemoto T (2009) Plasma Fibrinogen and D-dimer Concentrations are Associated with the presence of Abdominal Aortic Aneurysm: A Systematic Review and Meta-analysis. Eur J Vasc Endovasc Surg. 38:273-277

* Corresponding Author

[13] Freestone T, Turner R.J, Coady A, Higman D.J, Greenhalgh R.M, Powell J.T (1995) Inflammation and matrix metalloproteinases in the enlarging abdominal aortic aneurysm. Arterioscler Thromb Vasc Biol. 15(8):1145-51.

[14] McMillan W.D, Tamarina N.A, Cipollone M, Johnson D.A, Parker M.A, Pearce M.A, Pearce W.H (1997) Size matters: the relationship between MMP-9 expression and aortic diameter. Circulation. 96(7):2228-32.

[15] Pyo R, Jason L.K, Shipley M, Curci J.A, Mao D, Ziporin S.J et al. (2000) Targeted disruption of matrix-metalloproteinase-9 (gelatinase B) suppresses development of experimental abdominal aoric aneurysms. J Clin Invest. 105:1641-9.

[16] Thompson R.W, Parks W.C. (1996) Role of matrix metalloproteinases in abdominal aortic aneurysms. Ann NY Acad Sci. 800:157-174.

[17] Newman K.M et al. (1994) Identification of matrix metalloproteinases 3 (stomelysin-1) and 9 (gelatinase B) in abdominal aortic aneurysms. Arterioscler Thromb. 14: 1315-1320.

[18] Hovsepian D.M, Ziporin S.J, Sakurai M.K, Lee J.K, Curci J.A, Thompson R.W (2000) Elevated plasma levels of matrix metalloproteinase-9 in patients with abdominal aortic aneurysms: a circulating marker of degenerative aneurysm disease. J Vasc Interv Radiol. 11(10):1345-52

[19] Petersen E, Wagberg F, Angquist K.A (2002) Proteolysis of the Abdominal Aortic Aneurysm Wall and the Association with Rupture. Eur J Vasc Endovasc Surg. 23:153-157.

[20] Hellenthal F.A.M.V.I et al. (2012) Plasma Levels of Matrix Metalloproteinase-9: A Possible Diagnostic Marker of Successful Endovascular Aneurysm Repair. Eur J Vasc Endovasc Surg. 43:171-172.

[21] Wilson W.R.W, Anderton M, Choke E.C, Dawson J, Loftus I.M, Thompson M.M (2008) Elevated Plasma MMP1 and MMP9 are Associated with Abdominal Aortic Aneurysm Rupture. Eur J Vasc Endovasc Surg. 35:580-584.

[22] Karlsson L, Bergqvist D, Lindback J, Parsson H (2009) Expansion of Small-diameter Abdominal Aortic Aneurysms is Not Reflected by the Release of Inflammatory Mediators IL-6, MMP-9 and CRP in Plasma. Eur J Vasc Endovasc Surg. 37:420-424.

[23] Vega de Ceniga M, Esteban M, Quintana J.M, Barba A, Estallo L, De la Fuente N, Viviens B, Martin-Ventura J.L (2009) Search for Serum Biomarkers Associated with Abdominal Aortic Aneurysm Growth- A Pilot Study. Eur J Vasc Endovasc Surg. 37:297-299.

[24] Al-Barjas H.S, Ariens R, Grant P, Scott J.A (2006) Raised plasma fibrinogen concentration in patients with abdominal aortic aneurysm. Angiology. 57:607-14.

[25] Lindholt J.S et al. (2011) Insulin-like Growth Factor I- A Novel Biomarker of Abdominal Aortic Aneurysms. Eur J Vasc Endovasc Surg. 42:560-562.

[26] Urbonavicius S, Urbonaviciene G, Honore B, Henneberg E.W, Vorum H, Lindholt J.S (2008) Potential Circulating Biomarkers for Abdominal Aortic Aneurysm Expansion and Rupture – a Systematic Review. Eur J Vasc Endovasc Surg. 36:273-280.

[27] Parodi J.C, Palmaz J.C, Barone H.D (1991) Transfemoral intraluminal graft implantation for abdominal aortic aneurysms. Ann Vasc Surg. 5:496.

[28] Parodi J.C (1995) Endovascular repair of abdominal aortic aneurysms. In: Chuter T, Donayre C.E, White R.A, editors. Endoluminal Vascular Prostheses. Brown and Company. pp.37-55.

[29] Matsumura J.S, Brewster D.C, Makaroun M, Naftel D.C (2003) A multicenter controlled clinical trial of open versus endovascular treatment of abdominal aortic aneurysm. Journal of Vascular Surgery. 37:262-271.

[30] Goncalves F.B, Rouwet E.V, Metz R, Hendriks J.M, Vrancken Peeters M.P, Muhs B.E, Verhagen H.J (2010) Device-specific outcomes after endovascular abdominal aortic aneurysm repair. J Cardiovasc Surg. 51:515-531.

[31] Chaikof E.L, Brewster D.C, Dalman R.L, Makaroun M, Illig K.A, Sicard G.A, Timaran C.H, Upchurch Jr G.R, Veith F.J (2009) SVS practice guidelines for the care of patients with abdominal aortic aneurysm: Executive summary. Journal of Vascular Surgery. 50:880-896.

[32] Mani K, Lees T, Beiles B, Jensen L.P, Venermo M, Simo G, Palombo D et al. (2011) Treatment of Abdominal Aortic Aneurysm in Nine Countries 2005-2009: A Vascunet Report. . Eur J Vasc Endovasc Surg. 42; 598-607.

[33] EVAR Trial Participants (2005) Endovascular aneurysm repair versus open repair in patients with abdominal aortic aneurysm (EVAR trial 1): randomised controlled trial. The Lancet. 365: 2179-86.

[34] Prinssen M, Verhoeven E.L, Buth J, Cuypers P.W, van Sambeek M.R, Balm R et al. (2004) A randomised trial comparing conventional and endovascular repair of abdominal aortic aneurysms. N Engl J Med. 351:1607-18.

[35] Aljabri B, Al Wahaibi K, Abner D, Mackenzie K.S, Corriveau M.M, Obrand D.I et al. (2006) Patient-reported quality of life after abdominal aortic aneurysm surgery: a prospective comparison of endovascular and open repair. J Vasc Surg. 44(6):1182-7.

[36] Schroeder T.V (2006) Registries on endovascular aortic aneurysm repair. Pitfalls and benefits. J Cardiovasc Surg. 47:55-59.

[37] Thomas S.M, Gaines P.A, Beard J.D (2001) Short-term (30 day) outcome of endovascular treatment of abdominal aortic aneurysm: results from the prospective Registry of Endovascular Treatment of Abdominal Aortic Aneurysm (RETA). Eur J Vasc Endovasc Surg. 21:57-64.

[38] Harris P.L, Vallabhanemi R, Desgranges P, Becquemin J.P, van Marrewijk C, Laheij R (2000) Incidence and risk factors of late rupture, conversion, and death after endovascular repair of infrarenal aortic aneurysms: The EUROSTAR experience. Journal of Vascular Surgery. 32:739-749.

[39] Lifeline Registry of EVAR Publications Committee (2005) Lifeline registry of endovascular aneurysm repair: Long-term primary outcome measures. Journal of Vascular Surgery. 42:1-10.

[40] Hobo R, Sybrandy J, Harris P.L, Buth J (2008) Endovascular repair of abdominal aortic aneurysms with concomitant common iliac artery aneurysm: outcome analysis of the EUROSTAR experience. Journal of Endovascular Therapy. 15:12-22.

[41] The EVAR trial participants (2004) Comparison of endovascular aneurysm repair with open repair in patients with abdominal aortic aneurysm (EVAR trial 1), 30-day operative mortality results: randomised controlled trial. The Lancet. 364:843-848.

[42] The EVAR trial participants (2005) Endovascular aneurysm repair and outcome in patients unfit for open repair of abdominal aortic aneurysm (EVAR trial 2): randomised controlled trial. The Lancet. 365:2187-2192.

[43] Beard J.D (2006) EVAR for fit patients: evidence from the randomised trials. In: Wyatt M.G, Watkinson A.F, editors. Endovascular Therapies- Current Evidence. United Kingdom: Shrewsbury.pp.29-36.

[44] Prinssen M, Buskens E, Blankensteijn J.D (2002) The Dutch Randomized Endovascular Aneurysm Management (DREAM) trial background, design and methods. J Cardiovasc Surg. 43:379-384.

[45] Blankensteijn J.D, de Jong S.E, Prinssen M, van der Ham A.C, Buth J (2005) Dutch Randomized Endovascular Aneurysm Management (DREAM) trial group: two-year results of a randomized trial comparing conventional and endovascular repair of abdominal aortic aneurysms. N Engl J Med. 352:2398-2405.

[46] Lederle F.A (2007) The veterans open versus endovascular repair (OVER) trial for AAA - what will it add to EVAR 1 and DREAM? In: Becquemin J.P, Alimi Y.S, editors. Controversies and Updates in Vascular Surgery 2007. Minerva Medica. pp.101-102.

[47] Moll F.L, Powell J.T, Fraedrich G, Verzini F, Haulon S, Waltham M , van Herwaarden J.A, Holt P.J.E, van Keulen J.W, Rantner B, Schlosser F.J.V, Setacci F, Ricco J.B (2011) Management of Abdominal Aortic Aneurysms Clinical Practice Guidelines of the European Society for Vascular Surgery. Eur J Vasc Endovasc Surg. 41; S1-S58.

[48] The UK Small Aneurysm Trial Participants (1998) Mortality results for randomised controlled trial of early elective surgery or ultrasonographic surveillance for small abdominal aortic aneurysms. The Lancet. 352:1649-55.

[49] Lederle F.A, Wilson S.E, Johnson G.R, Reinke D.B, Littooy F.N, Acher C.W et al. (2002) Aneurysm Detection and Management Veterans Affairs Cooperative Study Group. Immediate repair compared with surveillance of small abdominal aortic aneurysms.N Engl J Med. 346:1437-44.

[50] Cao P (2005) Comparison of surveillance vs aortic endografting for small aneurysm repair (CAESAR) trial: study design and progress. Eur J Vasc Endovasc Surg. 30:245-51.

[51] Ouriel K (2009) The pivotal study: a randomised comparison of endovascular repair versus surveillance in patients with smaller abdominal aortic aneurysms. J Vasc Surg. 49: 266-9.

[52] Powell J.T, Brown L.C, Forbes J.F, Fowkes F.G, Greenhalgh R.M, Ruckley C.V et al. (2007) Final 12-year follow-up of surgery versus surveillance in the uk small aneurysm trial. Br J Surg. 94: 702-8.

[53] Ballard D.J, Filardo G, Fowkes G, Powell J.T (2008) Surgery for small asymptomatic abdominal aortic aneurysms. Cochrane Database Syst Rev. CD001835.

[54] Argenteri A, Curci R, Bianchi G, Orlandi M, de Amicis P (2009) Morphology and classifications of abdominal aortic aneurysms. In: Setacci C, Gasparini D, Reimers B, Cremonesi A, Rossi P.T, editors. Aortic Surgery New Developments and Perspectives. Minerva Medica. pp. 215-225.

[55] Raithel D, Qu L, Hetzel G (2007) Adapting the graft to the patient's anatomy: is this a way of solving all the problems? In: Becquemin J.P, Alimi Y.S, editors. Controversies and Updates in Vascular Surgery 2007. Minerva Medica. pp.150-156.

[56] Chisci E, De Donato G, Setacci F, Sirignano P, Galzerano G, Cappelli A, Palasciano G, Setacci C (2009) Standard elective endovascular aortic aneurysm repair (EVAR). In: Setacci C, Gasparini D, Reimers B, Cremonesi A, Rossi P.T, editors. Aortic Surgery New Developments and Perspectives. Minerva Medica. pp.227-147.

[57] Brennan J, Gambardella I (2006) Aortic stent grafts: current availability and applicability. In: Wyatt M.G, Watkinson A.F, editors. Endovascular Therapies. tfm Publishing Ltd. pp.1-11.

[58] Freyrie A, Testi G, Faggioli G, Gargiulio M, Giovanetti F, Serra C, Stella A (2010) Ring-stents supported infrarenal aortic endografts fits well in abdominal aortic aneurysms with tortuous anatomy. J Cardiovasc Surg. 51:467-474.

[59] Ghotbi R, Sotiriou A, Mansur R (2010) New results with 100 Excluder cases. J Cardiovasc Surg. 51:475-480.

[60] Bockler D, Fitridge R, Wolf Y, Hayes P, Silveira P.G, Numan F, Riambau V (2010) Rationale and design of the Endurant Stent Graft Natural Selection Global Postmarket Registry (ENGAGE): interim analysis at 30 days of the first 180 patients enrolled. J Cardiovasc Surg. 51:481-491.

[61] Becquemin J.P, Aksoy M, Marzelle J, Roudot-Thoraval F, Desgranges P, Allaire E, Kobeiter H (2008) Abdominal aortic aneurysm sac behavior following Cook Zenith graft implantation: a five-year follow-up assessment of 212 cases. J Cardiovasc Surg. 49:199-206.

[62] Krajcer Z, Gregoric I (2010) Totally percutaneous aortic aneurysm repair: methods and outcomes using the fully integrated IntuiTrak Endovascular System. J Cardiovasc Surg. 51:493-501.

[63] Moulakakis K.G, Avgerinos E.D, Giannakopoulos T, Papapetrou A, Brountzos E.N, Liapis C.D (2010) Current knowledge on E-vita abdominal endograft. J Cardiovasc Surg. 51:533-538.

[64] Stableford J.A, Maldonado T.S, Berland T, Kim B, Adelman M.A, Pachter H.L, Mussa F (2009) Endograft infection after EVAR. Endovascular Today. 8:35-38.

[65] Franks S.C, Sutton A.J, Bown M.J, Sayers R.D (2007) Systematic review and meta-analysis of 12 years of endovascular abdominal aortic aneurysm repair. Eur J Vasc Endovasc Surg. 33:154-171.

[66] Akkersdijk G.J, Prinssen M, Blankensteijn J.D (2004) The impact of endovascular treatment on in-hospital mortality following non-ruptured AAA repair over a decade: a population based study on 16446 patients. Eur J Vasc Endovasc Surg. 28:41-46.

[67] Gleason T.G (2009) Endoleaks after endovascular aortic stent-grafting: impact, diagnosis and management. Semin Thorac Cardiovasc Surg. 21:363-372.

[68] White G.H, Yu W, May J et al. (1997) Endoleak as a complication of endoluminal grafting of abdominal aortic aneurysms: classification, incidence, diagnosis and management. J Endovasc Surg. 4:152-168.

[69] Ricotta II J, Malgor R.D, Oderich G.S (2009) Traitement endovasculaire des anevrysmes de l'aorte abdominale: 1ere partie. Annales de Chirurgie Vasculaire. 23:864-878.

[70] van Keulen J.W, van Prehn J, Prokop M, Moll F.L, van Herwaarden J.A (2009) Potential value of aneurysm sac volume measurements in addition to diameter measurements after endovascular aneurysm repair. Journal of Endovascular Therapy. 16:506-513.

[71] Wolf Y.G, Tillich M, Lee A, Fogarty T.J, Zarins C.K, Rubin G.D (2002) Changes in aneurysm volume after endovascular repair of abdominal aortic aneurysm. Journal of Vascular Surgery. 36:305-309.

[72] Qu L, Raithel D (2008) Experience with the Endologix Powerlink endograft in endovascular repair of abdominal aortic aneurysms with short and angulated necks. Perspectives in Vascular Surgery and Endovascular Therapy. 20:158-166.

[73] Droc I, Raithel D, Pinte F, Nita D, Deaconu S, Popovici A, Molnar F, Finichi R, Candea B, Goleanu V (2008) Abdominal aortic aneurisms treatment - new devices for endovascular treatment. Romanian Journal of Cardiovascular Surgery. 7:235-242.

[74] Harkin D.W, Dillon M, Blair P.H, Ellis P.K, Kee F (2007) Endovascular ruptured abdominal aortic aneurysm repair (EVRAR): a systematic review. Eur J Vasc Endovasc Surg. 34:673-681.

[75] Richards T, Goode S.D, Hinchliffe R, Altaf N, MacSweeney S, Braithwaite B (2009) The importance of anatomical suitability and fitness for the outcome of endovascular repair of ruptured abdominal aortic aneurysm. Eur J Vasc Endovasc Surg. 38:285-290.

[76] Perrott S, Puckridge P.J, Foreman R.K, Russell D.A, Spark J.I (2010) Anatomical suitability for endovascular AAA repair may affect outcomes following rupture. Eur J Vasc Endovasc Surg. 40:186-190.

[77] Veith F.J, Cayne N (2009) Endovascular repair for ruptured abdominal aortic aneurysms: why the results vary. Vascular Disease Management. 6:165-170.

[78] Amiot S, Haulon S, Becquemin J.P, Magnan P.E, Lermusiaux P, Goueffic Y, Jean-Baptiste E, Cochennec F, Favre J.P (2010) Fenestrated endovascular grafting: the french multicentre experience. Eur J Vasc Endovasc Surg. 39:537-544.

[79] Greenberg R.K, Sternbergh W.C, Makaroun M, Ohki T, Chuter T, Bharadwaj P, Saunders A (2009) Intermediate results of a United States multicenter trial of fenestrated endograft repair for juxtarenal abdominal aortic aneurysms. Journal of Vascular Surgery. 50:730-737.

[80] O'Neill S, Greenberg R.K, Haddad F, Resch T, Sereika J, Katz E (2006) A prospective analysis of fenestrated endovascular grafting: intermediate-term outcome. Eur J Vasc Endovasc Surg. 32:115-123.

[81] Budde R.P.J, Huo F, Cramer M.J.M, Doevendans P.A, Bots M.L, Moll F.L, Prokop M (2010) Simultaneous aortic and coronary assessment in abdominal aortic aneurysm patients by thoraco-abdominal 64-detector-row CT angiography: estimate of the impact on preoperative management: a pilot study. Eur J Vasc Endovasc Surg. 40:196-201.

[82] Jean-Baptiste E, Hassen-Khodja R, Bouillanne P.J, Haudebourg P, Declemy S, Batt M (2007) Endovascular repair of infrarenal abdominal aortic aneurysms in high-risk-surgical patients. Eur J Vasc Endovasc Surg. 34:145-151.

[83] Steinmetz E, Abello N, Kretz B, Gauthier E, Bouchot O, Brenot R (2010) Analysis of outcome after using high-risk criteria selection to surgery versus endovascular repair in the modern era of abdominal aortic aneurysm treatment. Eur J Vasc Endovasc Surg. 39:403-409.

[84] Malkawi A.H, Hinchliffe R.J, Holt P.J, Loftus I.M, Thompson M.M (2010) Percutaneous access for endovascular aneurysm repair: a systematic review. Eur J Vasc Endovasc Surg. 39:676-682.

[85] Raman V.K, Karmarkar P.V, Guttman M.A et al. (2005) Real-time magnetic resonance-guided endovascular repair of experimental abdominal aortic aneurysm in swine. J Am Coll Cardiol. 45:2069-2077.

Permissions

The contributors of this book come from diverse backgrounds, making this book a truly international effort. This book will bring forth new frontiers with its revolutionizing research information and detailed analysis of the nascent developments around the world.

We would like to thank Yasuo Murai, for lending his expertise to make the book truly unique. He has played a crucial role in the development of this book. Without his invaluable contribution this book wouldn't have been possible. He has made vital efforts to compile up to date information on the varied aspects of this subject to make this book a valuable addition to the collection of many professionals and students.

This book was conceptualized with the vision of imparting up-to-date information and advanced data in this field. To ensure the same, a matchless editorial board was set up. Every individual on the board went through rigorous rounds of assessment to prove their worth. After which they invested a large part of their time researching and compiling the most relevant data for our readers. Conferences and sessions were held from time to time between the editorial board and the contributing authors to present the data in the most comprehensible form. The editorial team has worked tirelessly to provide valuable and valid information to help people across the globe.

Every chapter published in this book has been scrutinized by our experts. Their significance has been extensively debated. The topics covered herein carry significant findings which will fuel the growth of the discipline. They may even be implemented as practical applications or may be referred to as a beginning point for another development. Chapters in this book were first published by InTech; hereby published with permission under the Creative Commons Attribution License or equivalent.

The editorial board has been involved in producing this book since its inception. They have spent rigorous hours researching and exploring the diverse topics which have resulted in the successful publishing of this book. They have passed on their knowledge of decades through this book. To expedite this challenging task, the publisher supported the team at every step. A small team of assistant editors was also appointed to further simplify the editing procedure and attain best results for the readers.

Our editorial team has been hand-picked from every corner of the world. Their multi-ethnicity adds dynamic inputs to the discussions which result in innovative outcomes. These outcomes are then further discussed with the researchers and contributors who give their valuable feedback and opinion regarding the same. The feedback is then collaborated with the researches and they are edited in a comprehensive manner to aid the understanding of the subject.

Apart from the editorial board, the designing team has also invested a significant amount of their time in understanding the subject and creating the most relevant covers. They scrutinized every image to scout for the most suitable representation of the subject and create an appropriate cover for the book.

The publishing team has been involved in this book since its early stages. They were actively engaged in every process, be it collecting the data, connecting with the contributors or procuring relevant information. The team has been an ardent support to the editorial, designing and production team. Their endless efforts to recruit the best for this project, has resulted in the accomplishment of this book. They are a veteran in the field of academics and their pool of knowledge is as vast as their experience in printing. Their expertise and guidance has proved useful at every step. Their uncompromising quality standards have made this book an exceptional effort. Their encouragement from time to time has been an inspiration for everyone.

The publisher and the editorial board hope that this book will prove to be a valuable piece of knowledge for researchers, students, practitioners and scholars across the globe.

List of Contributors

Simona Celi
Institute of Clinical Physiology National Research Council IFC-CNR, Massa Fondazione Toscana CNR "G. Monasterio", Heart Hospital, Massa, Italy

Sergio Berti
Fondazione Toscana CNR "G. Monasterio", Heart Hospital, Massa, Italy

Ivanilson Alves de Oliveira
Neuroradiology, Experimental Medicine Laboratory, Universidade Federal de Sergipe-UFS, Brazil

Katarzyna Socha and Maria H. Borawska
Department of Bromatology, Medical University of Bialystok, Poland

Krzysztof Siemianowicz
Medical University of Silesia, Department of Biochemistry, Poland

Guillermo Vilalta and Félix Nieto
Mechanical Engineering Division, CARTIF Centro Tecnológico, Boecillo (Valladolid), Spain

Enrique San Norberto and Carlos Vaquero
Angiology and Vascular Surgery Service, University and Clinic Hospital of Valladolid, Valladolid, Spain

María Ángeles Pérez
ITAP Institute, University of Valladolid, Valladolid, Spain

José A. Vilalta
Industrial Engineering Department, Polytechnical University of Havana, Havana, 19340, Cuba

Ana Mladenovic and Zeljko Markovic
Faculty of Medicine Belgrade University, Clinical Center of Serbia, Center of Radiology and Magnetic Resonance, Serbia

Sandra Grujicic-Sipetic
Institute of Epidemiology Faculty of Medicine Belgrade University, Serbia

Hideki Hyodoh
Department of Radiology, Sapporo Medical University, Sapporo, Japan

Efstratios Georgakarakos, George S. Georgiadis, Konstantinos C. Kapoulas, Evagelos Nikolopoulos and Miltos Lazarides
"Democritus" University of Thrace Medical School, Alexandroupolis, Greece

Antonios Xenakis
Fluids Section, School of Mechanical Engineering, National Technical University of Athens, Athens, Greece

Ahmad Alsheikhly
Hamad Medical Corporation, Doha, Qatar

Ionel Droc and Blanca Calinescu
Cardiovascular Surgery Department, Army's Clinic Center for Cardiovascular Diseases, Bucharest, Romania

Dieter Raithel
Klinikum Nürnberg Sud, Nürnberg, Germany